Hospital Survival

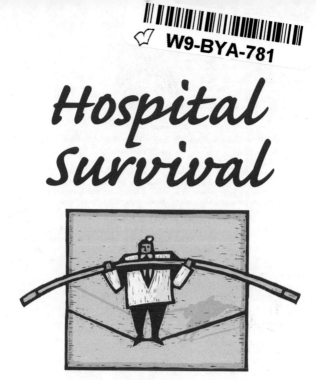

Lessons Learned in Medical Training

GRANT COOPER, M.D.

Resident

Department of Physical Medicine and Rehabilitation
New York–Presbyterian Hospital
The University Hospital of Columbia and Cornell
New York, New York

Wolters Kluwer | Lippincott Williams & Wilkins
Health

Philadelphia • Baltimore • New York • London
Buenos Aires • Hong Kong • Sydney • Tokyo

Acquisitions Editor: Donna M. Balado
Managing Editor: Kelly Horvath
Marketing Manager: Jennifer Kuklinski
Production Editor: Julie Montalbano
Designer: Doug Smock
Compositor: International Typesetting and Composition

9 8 7 6 5 4 3 2 1

Library of Congress Cataloging-in-Publication Data

Cooper, Grant, M.D.
   Hospital survival : lessons learned in medical training / Grant Cooper.
      p. ; cm.
   ISBN-13: 978-0-7817-7952-4
   1. Residents (Medicine)—Anecdotes. 2. Medical students—Anecdotes. 3. Clinical
medicine—Study and teaching—Anecdotes. 4. Hospital care—Anecdotes. I. Title.
   [DNLM: 1. Internship and Residency—Anecdotes. 2. Hospitals—Anecdotes. 3. Medical
Errors—prevention & control—Anecdotes. WX 203 C776h 2008]
   R840.C66 2008
   610.92—dc22

                                                                        2007009911

DISCLAIMER

   Care has been taken to confirm the accuracy of the information present and to describe generally accepted practices. However, the authors, editors, and publisher are not responsible for
errors or omissions or for any consequences from application of the information in this book
and make no warranty, expressed or implied, with respect to the currency, completeness, or
accuracy of the contents of the publication. Application of this information in a particular situation remains the professional responsibility of the practitioner; the clinical treatments
described and recommended may not be considered absolute and universal recommendations.

   The authors, editors, and publisher have exerted every effort to ensure that drug selection
and dosage set forth in this text are in accordance with the current recommendations and
practice at the time of publication. However, in view of ongoing research, changes in govern-
ment regulations, and the constant flow of information relating to drug therapy and drug
reactions, the reader is urged to check the package insert for each drug for any change in
indications and dosage and for added warnings and precautions. This is particularly important when the recommended agent is a new or infrequently employed drug.

   Some drugs and medical devices presented in this publication have Food and Drug
Administration (FDA) clearance for limited use in restricted research settings. It is the
responsibility of the health care provider to ascertain the FDA status of each drug or device
planned for use in their clinical practice.

To purchase additional copies of this book, call our customer service department at **(800)
638-3030** or fax orders to **(301) 223-2320.** International customers should call **(301) 223-2300.**

Visit Lippincott Williams & Wilkins on the Internet: *http://www.lww.com.* Lippincott Williams &
Wilkins customer service representatives are available from 8:30 am to 6:00 pm, EST.

Preface

Some of my favorite times in residency have been sitting around the call room with my colleagues gossiping about the crazy, nonsensical, stupid, and all too human things we, yes *we*, have done. I don't particularly like gossip—but don't knock it completely. If you listen closely enough, you may find some underlying wisdom. I'll give you an example. In medical school, one of the top students in my class, and a friend of mine, had a particularly unfortunate experience. His resident had given him the unenviable task of performing a guaiac on a patient with severe Crohn's disease and history of a GI bleed. He related the following story:

> It was the end of the day, and already dark outside. I went into the patient's room but didn't want to turn on all of the lights because she seemed to have already fallen asleep. I gently woke her up and introduced myself in the dim light. I told her what I needed to do, did the rectal quickly and put the drops on. There was no bleeding, so I told the patient: "Good news. You're not bleeding into your gut."
>
> She looked surprised and said, "You can tell that from checking down there?"
>
> "Yes," I told her, not really understanding yet.
>
> "You mean, it's connected?" she persisted, sitting up in bed.
>
> Then I realized what I had done. My face turned bright, bright red. I told her we would check again in a little while just

to be sure. I abruptly turned around and left. Later, I couldn't force myself to go back into her room, so I asked the other medical student on the rotation to do the guaiac for me as a favor, this time in the correct anatomic cavity.

This book mentions no real names and these stories are not meant to embarrass anyone. On the contrary, if anything, I hope that this book makes us feel a little less embarrassed about our own mistakes. We are all human, and we all have made, or will make, mistakes that in retrospect seem obvious. Even your attending, the one who is so sure of herself; the chief resident who never makes a mistake or fails to remind you when you do; or the austere department chair has had at least one day when he or she could relate to "guaiac boy." It happens to all of us. The important thing is to learn from it and move on. This book is dedicated to that premise. The advantage of the written word is that we can benefit from other people's misfortunes. We can learn from them the easy way . . . so hopefully, we won't have to always learn the hard way. Take guaiac boy, for example. What is the moral there?

The moral of guaiac boy: Take your time to make sure you can see what you're doing, for starters. Second, learn from what he did right. If the patient asks you why you did something, and you know you screwed up, consider your options. Come clean—always admirable and it's my first choice. Be mature and explain your mistake. This patient had a long history of Crohn's and a lot of fibrosis in the area in question. She would have understood if he had explained. While guaiac boy didn't come clean, he also didn't lose his cool or behave unprofessionally either. He didn't gasp, giggle, or cringe. He chose (probably because of embarrassment rather than honor) discretion—which sometimes could arguably be the better side of valor. Third, if possible, stay in there and do the job right. If guaiac boy had simply stayed put, explained his mistake, and repeated the test, this time in the correct cavity, it would have been over, and he would have felt better about himself. Also, he wouldn't have felt it necessary to ask the other medical student to go back and do it for him.

This is the book that I wish I had had when I started internship. I'll give you the scoop about what to absolutely do and not do. Might some of the stories in this book be urban legend? Absolutely. But many urban legends are born on a kernel of truth and are passed down for a reason. And many of these stories I know without a doubt are not legend—they are frightening, unbelievable, I-never-want-to-be-a-patient-in-a-hospital, fact. I hope you will enjoy and learn from them.

A final three notes before we get started:

First note—The lessons in this book are applicable to any medical student doing a clinical rotation, intern, or resident. The stories are almost all about interns because the events that accompany beginning, surviving, and thriving during that taxing year often make for the most colorful and dramatic anecdotes. As the voice of this book, I have also chosen to address my comments to the developing intern. But, to be sure, these are lessons that are intended for students and residents as well.

Second note—The lessons are presented as a list of "Do's" and "Don'ts." Almost every "Do" or "Don't" is followed by an anecdote about someone who didn't or did. Friends and colleagues, as well as very helpful professional reviewers, who have read the first drafts of this book suggested that while some of the Do's and Don'ts listed are less obvious, some of them seem more obvious to them. Almost *too* obvious. Indeed, hopefully, when you read the Don'ts, you'll think, "I would never do that, anyway." Similarly, when you read the Do's, you will hopefully say to yourself, "Of course I would do that." The more obvious Do's and Don'ts are not meant to insult your intelligence or common sense or to suggest you would have done otherwise without the aid of this book. Simply keep in mind that with the long hours and increased stresses of internship, common sense is often the first casualty. And remember that, to get into this book, at least one intern (or resident) had to make the mistake in the first place. So, to at least one doctor, the Do or Don't was not that obvious. This book presents the cases of these unfortunates so that you hear their stories and, ideally, learn from them.

Third note—The language that I use in this book is on the stronger side. *Do this. Don't do that.* If you aren't already tired of authority figures telling you what to do and not do, by the end of internship you probably will be. This book is not meant to add to the burden of your responsibilities. Rather, it is aimed at helping you navigate the waters and particularly the high tides. I use the strong language because I think it sticks in people's heads better, is more entertaining, and because it is the way that I wish I had been talked to and guided when I was an intern. As my father-in-law says, "Don't bull#$&@ me. Just give me the facts."

I offer two brief anecdotes to similar effect:

My older brother and I were throwing a baseball together out-side. I was a freshman and he was a senior in high school. We were getting ready for the new season. He was throwing the ball to me much harder than I was used to, and my hand was throbbing. My brother, Aaron, noted my discomfort. "If you want to get good and play varsity, you have to be able to han-dle this." That was all he needed to tell me. My hand still hurt, but I stopped noticing.

A few years later, I was a returning varsity player in the middle of soccer preseason. We had broken up into two teams. The younger players were competing for a spot on varsity. One of the younger players was a friend of mine. A ball landed between us in the middle of the scrimmage. We both went for the ball and collided. I sent him to the ground, took the ball, and dribbled up the field. I could hear him complaining behind me that I had fouled him. When the play was over, I ran back to him and walked with him for a second. "This is varsity," I told him. "It's more physical. If you want to play here, you have to toughen up and be okay with the contact." He became one of the toughest players on our team.

This is internship. You're a doctor now. You are still learning, but your patients are *your* patients. The incre-mental jump in responsibility and expectations from student to intern is tremendous. Take a moment. Take a breath. In a moment of calm, read through this book and let it help you become the toughest, smartest, most competent intern on your team.

Acknowledgments

This book would not have been possible without the help, love, and support of my wife, Ana. When discussing what was the secret to becoming a successful author, the prolific Stephen Ambrose once wrote, "Marry an English major." I can only dream of being as accomplished a writer as Mr. Ambrose, however it tickles me that I share a common experience with him. Just as he leaned on and needed his wife, Moira, for his work, I rely on mine. Ana's endless enthusiasm, understanding, encouragement, and good humor create the stimulating environment in which I write. From such a place, I believe positive results are inevitable.

I would like to thank my publisher, Lippincott Williams & Wilkins. I extend a special thank you to Donna Balado. As senior acquisitions editor, Donna's vision, drive, and willingness to try something new allowed this book to become a reality. Thank you to Kelly Horvath who, as development editor, provided invaluable help with the formation of this book.

I would also like to say thank you to my brother-in-law Viktor for reminding me that no matter how hard I may work, someone is working harder. Thank you, too, to my parents-in-law Dragomir and Ljubica. From blocks to books, my parents' support and love provide the foundation for all that I do. I extend an extra thanks to my mom, for her tireless reading and re-reading of this manuscript, and for all of her helpful insights and encouragement. I would like to thank my brothers, sister-in-law, and nephews. A final thank you, too, to Mark, for reminding me to lead with a "5" or maybe a "7," but to keep the "1" close at hand. It all works out in the end if you keep a tall glass of chocolate milk and a bowl of macaroni and cheese on the table.

Contents

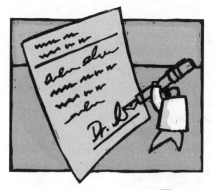

Documenting: Do's and Don'ts

👍 BE CAREFUL AND ACCURATE WHEN WRITING ORDERS

Confusing "units" with "cc" or "mg" when writing orders might seem to be merely an "academic" mistake. After all, everyone knows what you mean, right? Not necessarily! When you become an intern and start writing orders for patients, you have to get it right. Consider the following experience:

My wife, who is also a doctor, recalls the story of an intern in a busy university hospital who, during his first few weeks on the floors, wrote precisely for 10 cc of insulin for one of his patients. He knew better than to write that order. No one gets 10 cc of insulin. You get 10 units of insulin. He shouldn't have written it.

The nurse should have caught the mistake. But, she didn't. The pharmacy should have flagged it. But, they didn't. So the patient got 10 cc of insulin and subsequently went into a coma. It was awful for the patient, his family, and the intern. The intern, after all, was seriously overworked. His internship program was known to be "old school," hardcore, and they didn't think the work hour rules (which were in place when he was an intern) applied to them. So the intern was tired, very tired. He meant no harm. It was a mistake. But it was a mistake that was severely detrimental to the patient and cost the intern his job.

LESSON LEARNED

The moral of this story is clear. Without belaboring the point, it is important to pause and consider that you are passing into a new phase of life. The expectation bar is higher, and failure to reach those expectations will only be tolerated so far. Even when you're tired; even when you realize that the world isn't fair and you really do need sleep; even when you just want to go home—perhaps especially then—you really do need to check and double check your work, particularly your orders. If you make a mistake in a note, that can be forgiven. If you make a mistake with patient care, the consequences may be too severe to be forgiven. Many hospitals have instituted computer orders, likely resulting in fewer errors due to grossly incorrect units or dosages. But even computerized orders can be wrong. So be careful.

Legend has it that when Roman engineers constructed their great arches, the chief engineer would stand beneath the arch as the temporary buttresses and supporting scaffolding were removed for the first time.

That way, if the work turned out shoddy in any way, and the arch collapsed, the engineer would not live to build another one. The engineer's work was important not only to his reputation but also, in a stark and immediate sense, to his life. It is a relevant story to keep in the back of your mind when you are treating your patients. Your life might not hang in the balance of your orders, but always remember that your patient's does.

👍 CONFIRM ALL INFORMATION IN A PATIENT'S CHART

Copying incorrect information out of the patient's chart happens all the time. One doctor writes down that the patient has crackles in his lungs, and every subsequent doctor who writes in the chart records the exact same information. Never mind that the patient had no crackles to begin with or that the patient did have crackles but then received a diuretic and the crackles went away. Perhaps the first doctor writes down that the patient has a history of benign prostatic hypertrophy (BPH). Then, everyone copies that information. When one astute attending finally asks why the patient is not being treated for his BPH, it is discovered that he never had a history of BPH after all. Or, worse, a doctor sees that the patient has "BPH" but is not on any treatment, so he or she starts him on a medication.

Don't copy information from the chart without independently verifying it. I know it's burdensome. Your time is limited, and it is difficult to have to confirm everything. In addition, patients sometimes resent repeating the same information over and over. To some extent, you have to rely on your colleagues for help, including information. But, when it comes to your patients, you really should ask for yourself. You can streamline the process by getting as much information from the chart as possible and retelling patients what you think you know about them. Then, let the patient correct you. "No, no doc, I don't have any problem with my urine." Or, the patient might say, "Yes, but doc, the real problem is in my stomach." Make sure to confirm your information with the patient. And when it comes to lab results, check them yourself, always. Consider the following example:

You have a patient on your service who is being followed by neurology for Parkinson's. The neurology resident comes in early to round on her patients. She sees your patient and writes her note. She is primarily concerned with his Parkinson's, but to make her note billable for her attending, she has to include labs. So, she writes labs in her note. But she doesn't take the time to make sure that she recorded today's labs, or maybe she just copied the labs from yesterday from someone else's note.

An hour later, you come to see the patient. You are writing your note and are thankful to see the labs already recorded. This way, you don't have to log onto the computer to check for yourself; besides, the computers are in high demand, and you don't have time to wait. You copy the labs only to find out later in the day that the patient's labs for the day were not normal, and she needed to have her potassium replaced.

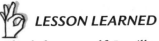 **LESSON LEARNED**

Check for yourself. It will cost you a few minutes, but will ultimately save you a big headache, not to mention ensure the safety of your patient.

4

DOCUMENT, DOCUMENT, AND DOCUMENT SOME MORE

In the hospital, if something isn't written in the chart, it didn't happen. You have to document every interaction you have with an attending, resident, or patient—or it didn't happen, period. Consider the following story told by an intern at a large urban hospital.

The patient was a 68-year-old female with a history of myocardial infarction (MI) 3 years prior. She was admitted to the hospital with fever and a cough and was found to have pneumonia. I was called to see her while on call because she was having chest discomfort and numbness and tingling in her hand. She described the chest discomfort as similar to the heartburn she was used to getting, but the hand symptoms were new. She had already tried some Maalox, which usually worked for her heartburn, but it hadn't helped. She said that her previous heart attack had felt different, more like stabbing chest pain. I still thought we had to rule out an MI, so I ordered labs and an EKG.

The EKG machine on our floor was broken. I had never encountered this before. The nurse said I should get another one from a different floor. I didn't know where to go so I called my resident. I told him everything that had happened, including the patient's symptoms and my physical exam. My resident told me that she was probably a little hypoxic, which would explain the numbness in her fingers.

"But her pulse ox is 96%," I reminded my resident.

He told me to give her some more Maalox and just go by the labs. I still remember the irritation in his voice when he said, "Don't worry about the EKG. Let the tech do it. Just put a note in the chart and come help me in the ER. We have three admissions and I'm all alone here. We'll check your lady's labs later. She'll be fine."

5

I didn't feel comfortable leaving my patient with her heartburn and numb/tingling fingers. But I was only in my second month of internship and still getting the hang of things. My resident was in his third year and very confident in his abilities. It probably was just heartburn, I told myself.

I ordered the labs STAT and told the nurse to give her some more Maalox and that I would be in the ER. The nurse barely acknowledged me and went about her business.

I ran down to the ER and started with the admissions. Periodically, I checked the computer to see if my patient's labs were back. One hour passed, then two, then three. When we were finished with the admissions, I told my resident the labs still weren't back. He told me, "If they haven't called back about her, then I'm sure she's fine. Don't worry about it. Come on, we have to go check on those other two patients on Blue 9."

"I'll meet you there. I just want to make sure the labs actually got drawn and the EKG was done." I went to my patient's room and found her in the same condition as I had left her. The Maalox hadn't helped, but she was comforted to know that we weren't worried.

"No, no one has come to take my blood or anything else," she responded when I asked her. "Should they have?"

"It's okay," I told her, "I'll take it now." We had ancillary staff that was supposed to do the blood draws, but sometimes they could be very slow. I drew the blood and sent it to the lab. There was still no EKG machine to be found so I asked the nurse to page the tech again. Then I went to join my resident and help with our other patients.

The labs came back for my patient about the same time that the nurse called me and told me that her pain had gotten worse. I looked on the screen and gulped. Her troponin was over 5. She ended up going to the cardiac intensive care unit and was treated for a large infarction.

The next day the attending in the cardiac intensive care unit called my attending. My attending called me and demanded to know why I hadn't gotten an EKG as I said I was going to in my event note. I told him the whole story, including how my resident had told me not to bother. My attending then called in my resident—my resident. I was standing right next to him when he came to the floor and lied through his teeth. He told my attending and later my director that I never told him that the patient was having anything other than heartburn.

My resident said to my director, "I told Bryan over the phone that if all she was having was a little heartburn, then just give her some Maalox. Bryan never mentioned her cardiac history and if he had told me that she was having chest discomfort that had already not been relieved by Maalox and that she was also having hand symptoms, I would have demanded that he do the EKG immediately."

Listening to him, my mouth dropped. I told the attendings that he was either not remembering what happened correctly or else he was just plain lying. My director made things very clear for me in a way I will never forget. He said, "It's not in your note, Bryan. You never even mention talking to your senior resident in your note. If it's not in your note, it didn't happen, and we have to go with your resident's version of what happened. Next time, write down that you talked to your resident and what he said. Then you'll be covered. Since you didn't do that, you're responsible. It's that simple."

When we were outside, I confronted my resident. "You lied," I told him.

He shook his head. "Bryan, you have to learn to take responsibility for your actions. She was your patient."

"You are my senior and you told me not to do the EKG myself. You hung me out to dry."

7

"She was your patient. You should know how to work up chest pain. I'm going to lunch."

And that's how it was. That was my wake-up call to the real world.

LESSON LEARNED

Don't learn this lesson the hard way. Other stories I could list here would reveal attendings and residents agreeing on a course of action that later proves to be inappropriate and wrong. When the resident is grilled about why he chose the treatment, the resident says that he consulted the attending. But, the note does not reveal this, and the attending denies it or says that they only briefly discussed it. No matter how nice or friendly your coworkers seem, some of them, and you never know whom, can turn out to be real first-class jerks. Always protect yourself.

Document, document, and document some more. After seeing a patient and talking with your attending physician, get in the habit of writing "D/W attending, agrees with plan." If you disagree with your attending and think that something bad might happen, simply write something like "After discussing the patient's status, including X, Y, and Z, will place orders as per attending." You don't have to be nasty, and you should always try to avoid disparaging your colleagues. But, I do believe that you need to protect yourself. Enough bad stories are circulating of interns and residents getting burned to make me think that you must take this matter very seriously. It's easy to help bulletproof yourself against it. Simply, document. The same goes for a consultant telling you to do something over the phone. That's fine, but document it. If you don't document that it was the consultant's order to you, and something bad happens, the consultant may very well say that he or she didn't tell you to do it or didn't have all the facts. If you document that you spoke to pager #1234, that pager #1234 was told of the patient's status, and that he advised X, Y, and Z, you will be more protected than had you not.

None of us became physicians because we love paperwork. Most of us would prefer to stay as far away from filling out papers and worrying about documentation as possible. Get over this lack of interest. The sooner you accept the reality that documentation is crucial, the better off you'll be. Documentation isn't only important in covering yourself during internship, it's important during residency, fellowship, and when you're an attending. And it's not just about covering your a** (CYA); it will also prove to be important for reimbursements. So start the good habits now: Document, document, document.

KEEP YOUR COMPUTER PASSWORD PRIVATE

Don't give anyone your password to the computer. Remember to sign off the hospital computer when you're finished using it. The following occurred at an urban university hospital.

Norman was a good intern. He was conscientious and hard working, and he was always willing to lend a helping hand to another intern. When his friend Jack got locked out of the computer system, Norman naturally didn't hesitate to give Jack his username and password. After all, it helped Jack out and it also prevented Norman from having to put in all of Jack's orders. Besides, he trusted Jack enough.

9

More than a month later, Norman was surprised when he was called into the director's office. Norman had no idea what the meeting was about. The director and Norman got along well, but now her face was stern. "Norman," she began, "Do you know why you're here?"

Norman soon learned that someone had used his user-name and password to look up information about a famous athlete who had been in the hospital. The director believed Norman when he said he had not done it. After all, it just didn't seem like something he would do. "Did you give your pass-word to anyone else?" The director asked.

"Well, just Jack. But Jack wouldn't do that. Someone else must have gotten my information somehow."

Jack was brought in for questioning. He, too, denied having accessed any improper information. He did reveal, however, that he had given Norman's username and password to a medical student so that he could put in orders for himself. In turn, the medical student was brought in and questioned at length. Through it all, the student maintained that he had not accessed any of the information in question.

The director believed Norman. The president of the hospital and the disciplinary committee were said to have believed Norman. The hospital, however, was a large university hospital with lots of high-profile people, and it was cracking down on Health Insurance Portability and Accountability Act (HIPAA) violations. Norman was thus held accountable nonetheless, and he was used as an example. Norman was suspended from his internship.

LESSON LEARNED

The moral here is clear. You all know about HIPAA by this time. You are not permitted to access medical information if you are not taking care of the patient. If medical information about a high-profile person (or any person for that matter!) is accessed improperly, someone is likely to be held accountable. If the accessing was done with your username and password, you are that person unless someone else confesses. Even if the true guilty party does confess, you still may be held partly accountable for providing access.

You may have all the trust in the world for a fellow intern, resident, student, or other staff member. But, do you trust that person with your career? Make no mistake about it: If you give someone your username and password, in effect that is what you are doing. Don't do it. Not only should others not be writing orders under your username and password, they shouldn't be tempted with the opportunity to look up other people's information. There are so many ways that this situation can end up badly, why take the chance? To make the day a *little* more expedient? So you don't have to do a little more extra work? It's not worth it. Interns and residents sometimes do share passwords. I've seen it. This is like playing with fire. Make it a rule that it's not something you do and no one will get offended. If someone asks, just tell the person asking you that you don't feel comfortable sharing your password. That person will (or at least *should*) understand and respect you for your limits. If he or she doesn't— well, it's your license and your career you're looking out for in this instance, not theirs.

On another anecdotal note, when I was doing an inpatient rotation during residency at Columbia Presbyterian Hospital, a well-known person was in the hospital recovering from heart surgery. It was rumored, though I have no direct knowledge of this, that several people were put on suspension, including nurses and attending physicians (I never heard of a resident doing this) for looking up the famous patient's medical information. Ironically, although the famous person was admitted under a pseudonym, another patient in the hospital apparently had the same (real) name. So, people who looked up the famous person's name to investigate his blood work (why this is interesting to people in the first place is beyond me) actually ended up with the other patient's medical information.

MAKE SURE YOU ARE COMFORTABLE WRITING ORDERS

If you don't feel comfortable writing an order, don't write it. Do discuss the order with your senior resident and/or attending physician.

As an intern, you will get used to writing orders at other people's direction. They will tell you to order lab tests, MRIs, CTs, medications, etc. At some point, you may be instructed to write an order that you don't agree with and you think may even be harmful to the patient. If this should happen, I ask you to do two things. First, talk to the person directing you to write the order. Explain your position and reasoning. Second, if you have explained your reasoning and your senior resident or attending *still* insists that you write the order, I would strongly advise that you respectfully inform your senior resident or attending that you will not write it if you think it is dangerous to the patient. Consider the following story from an intern at an urban hospital.

During my second medicine floor rotation I was on the green unit, which was the busiest. I had a senior resident who was always telling me what to do. He had this method of giving me a page of paper during the day with a "To Do" list. He gave me and the other intern on our team these papers two or three times a day. If we didn't do something on the list, he would berate us, so we pretty much learned to just do whatever was on our paper. One time, he wrote that I should give Bactrim to one of my patients.

"Doesn't this patient have an allergy to sulfa drugs?" I asked him.

"No," he said, annoyed that I was questioning him. "Just do it. I don't want to be here until eight again. You and Dougherty need to be more efficient."

I nodded, but persisted. "Are you sure he's not allergic? I think I saw it in the chart. I'll double check."

"For crying out loud," his face was getting red, as it sometimes did. "It says 'allergy' but if you ask him what happens when he takes sulfa drugs, he'll tell you that his stomach gets upset. Is stomach upset a true allergy?"

I didn't answer. I was tired and frustrated, too, and he knew that I knew it wasn't a true allergy.

"Okay, then go do your work," he barked.

I went back to the chart and looked through it. Sure enough, when the patient was in his 20s, he had Stevens-Johnson syndrome as what they thought was a reaction to a sulfa medication. He didn't remember which sulfa drug he had taken. I called my resident and told him. There was silence on the other end of the line. I didn't know how he would react. Then, my resident apologized and thanked me for checking. He was refreshingly reasonable, for a change. I knew he was just overworked and overstressed and so was acting like a jerk. In this instance, he had gotten my patient

13

confused with someone else on the other intern's team. If I had written the order he had instructed, who knows what would have happened to the patient and what kind of trouble he and I might have gotten into.

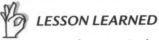 ## *LESSON LEARNED*

The point, of course, is that sometimes residents and attendings make mistakes. They ask you to write orders that aren't appropriate. In the above instance, if the intern hadn't caught the mistake, a nurse or the pharmacy might have caught it, but they might not have. A disastrous reaction could have ensued. If it did, not only would the patient suffer, but everyone involved (including and probably particularly the intern) would have gotten in trouble.

Realize that if you write an order, it is your MD or DO on the line. If you do find yourself in the position of writing an order that you might find questionable or might worry about, document the reason for the order, including who told you to write it and why.

If you explain why you think an order is inappropriate to the resident or attending, everyone will, or at least should, respect you for your desire to provide conscientious care for your patient and to understand why each order is being performed. Usually, discussing the order in question will either lead the attending or resident to change his or her mind or will convince you that there is a good reason for the order. In both cases, it is an extremely worthwhile exercise. Only rarely does a discussion of the order fail to resolve the issue.

Perhaps the following story, related by a resident in a community hospital, illustrates the point best.

My attending was a well-known professor. She had published many papers in her day, which was about a decade before I got to the hospital. She was an older woman and a generally anxious person. She liked having women on her service so we got along well, but I never felt completely comfortable with her. She was very intelligent, but when a patient was going downhill, she had a reputation for getting a little hysterical and not using good judgment. One day we had a patient who started dropping his oxygen saturation. He had a tender calf and we had a strong clinical suspicion for PE. We sent him down for a STAT CT angio and sure enough there was a large saddle embolus. My attending was almost frantic. She was pacing up and down the hall by the nursing station.

"Okay, okay," she said, coming next to me as I was getting ready to write orders in the chart. "He's going to the ICU. I just know it. Okay, well, start Lovenox 140 mg BID."

The patient weighed at most 70 kg. "Do you mean 70 mg BID?" I asked, knowing that was the correct dose.

"No, 140 mg. Write it now." She told me, tapping the chart with her index finger.

"But the dose for Lovenox in the treatment of a PE is 1 mg/kg BID, and he weighs less than 70 kg. I think we should probably give 70 mg BID."

"Listen," my attending told me, dismayed, "I've been doing this for a long time. This man has a large saddle embolus. If we don't anticoagulate more than usual, he'll tank. Everything we do isn't written in the books. Write for 140 mg. We don't have time to be screwing around, do we?"

I looked at my intern. Was she for real? I scanned my brain but had never heard of a dose that large. I was sure she was mistaken and not thinking clearly. "I can't write that dose," I told her. "He'll bleed."

15

My attending was visibly rattled. She wasn't used to residents telling her "No," and now some of the nurses' heads turned as they tuned in to the confrontation. My attending looked at my intern. My intern looked at me. I shook my head. "Look," I said to the attending. "Let's give 70 mg now and see how he does. We can always give more later."

My attending threw her pen on the counter. I still remember the look in her eyes. "Fine," she snapped and then stormed off.

Looking back, I think she was just happy to use a pretense to get off the floor and away from the crashing patient. We gave the appropriate dose. I called another attending I knew and ran the whole story by her. She completely agreed with me, so I felt better about the interaction. It was true that not everything we do in the hospital is written in books or backed by clear research, but I had never heard of such a high dose of Lovenox. The attending retired the next year, which I think made everyone breathe a little easier.

LESSON LEARNED

If the resident in the above example had written such a large and indefensible dose of Lovenox, she and the attending would have been held responsible if and when the patient bled. Of course, the above story is from a resident, but it could just as easily have been an intern. With less experience, it takes that much more self-composure for you, as an intern, to question orders—but you must do it nonetheless if you think the order is in error. In some instances, you may be the last line of defense against an egregious medical mistake.

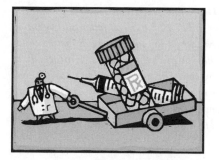

Chapter 2

Wards: Do's and Don'ts

👍 DON'T TOUCH ANYTHING YOU CAN'T IDENTIFY

When you become an intern, suddenly you're a doctor. People, especially patients, expect you to know things. Not only that, but *you* want to know things. You want to meet your patients', colleagues', and supervisors' expectations, and, importantly, your own. But if you see something and don't know what it is or how to handle it, don't touch it. The following story bears a harsh reminder of this necessity.

> When I was an intern, there was a family practice intern at our sister hospital who made a tragic mistake. A baby girl had come to the hospital suffering from an asthmatic attack. The patient—the baby girl—was stabilized, doing well, and

receiving oxygen. The family practice intern noticed that the tube connecting the child's IV fluids had fallen out. Wanting to be helpful, he reattached the tube for fluids for the child. The problem was that it wasn't the fluids he "reattached" to the IV. It was the oxygen. The tubing shouldn't have fit, but it did. The result was an air embolus that went straight into the child's lungs and killed her soon after. The intern didn't have to be fired. He quit, and last I heard he was still in therapy.

 LESSON LEARNED

In the emergency room and in the hospital in general, there are a lot of tubes, wires, and other gadgets lying around, beeping, and performing various functions. As you spend more time in the hospital, these sights and sounds will become second nature. The scene of so many tubes won't be confusing. It will be routine. You'll know which tube is the IV and where it should be connected. You'll know which tube is for the Foley, etc. If you don't know what should be connected or how to change the rate of a medication on an IV, don't do it yourself. Get someone to help you. No one expects you to know everything when you start—so ask! As the years progress, you may find it harder and harder to claim ignorance. Start asking questions early and often. No one can or should fault you for asking the question. Your patients, and you, will thank you. Incidentally, because of that unfortunate but well-intentioned intern, that hospital changed the tubing so that the oxygen and IV are no longer compatible. But, a million mistakes can be made if you don't know what you're doing. Since you don't know what you're doing when you start, stop and ask. A small step may avoid a huge mistake, and people will respect you for wanting to be careful.

👍 BE EXTREMELY CAREFUL AROUND NEEDLES

This is one of those obvious reminders that you just can't hear enough. Needles are dangerous. You have been taught how to handle them, but people still get sloppy when handling them becomes routine. We can all benefit from the stories of those who have been a little careless or just plain unlucky. Let their experiences remind you to be extra careful.

I'm the first medical doctor in my immediate family, so I admit that I didn't quite understand what I was getting myself into. Of course, going to medical school, I realized I was choosing a career in which I would be around a lot of sick people, including some with infectious diseases. I realized I would be exposed to various viruses, airborne and otherwise. I was prepared for this, and I also understood that I would be participating in operations, drawing blood, and placing IVs, but somehow I did not anticipate the amount of exposure or the amount of danger that all of this would entail.

I have to believe that by now you have experienced, seen, or heard your own horror stories with needle sticks. Consider the following story that happened in a small urban hospital. The voice is that of an intern in ob/gyn.

It was after dawn and we were doing our fourth straight C-section. I could barely keep my eyes open, and I was pretty much just retracting. I could tell that the attending was tired, too. The patient was a 15-year-old indigent female who had not received any prenatal care. Somewhere in the middle of the C-section, I felt a searing cut across the top of my thumb.

"Ouch," I said, immediately waking up. "I got cut." We didn't know her HIV or hepatitis status, which was the next thought that raced through my head. She was certainly at risk. What was her status?

"No," the attending told me, "you're fine. You didn't get cut."

I couldn't believe what I heard. "Yes, I did. I felt it. I got cut." From where I was standing, I couldn't see my hand, but I could certainly feel what had happened.

"Don't stop retracting. You're okay. We're almost done."

"I'm letting go," I told the attending. "Jody, put your hand here and hold." The medical student hesitantly did as I instructed. I felt bad asking her, but I had to get out of there. I looked at my hand and saw blood oozing out of the glove.

I went straight to the emergency room. They told me I had to go to occupational health. At occupational health, I met with the on-call counselor and she discussed my options with me. I could start antiretroviral therapy, which carried with it several severe potential side effects such as pancreatitis and kidney stones, or I could take my chances and ask the woman to get herself tested. They took my blood to get my baseline status for HIV and hepatitis.

The whole process, from leaving the OR to deciding not to start the antiretroviral therapy took about three hours. When I came back to the floor, the chief resident was rounding with the residents and interns.

"Where were you?" the chief resident asked me.

"Didn't you hear what happened? I just got back from occupational health."

"You mean you haven't rounded on any of your patients?"

"No, I haven't."

The chief stared at me, through me. She looked at me like I didn't exist, or shouldn't have existed. "If you have to go to the doctor, do it on your own time. You have patients and responsibilities here. Don't you care about them?!"

This was not a sincere question and I didn't respond.

For five excruciating days, I tried to get consent from the patient (which was difficult in its own right), waited for the labs to come back, and pondered my fate. She turned out to be negative for HIV and hepatitis B and C. I received zero sympathy from my residents and attendings. The other interns looked at me with a mixture of empathy and fear, realizing it could easily happen to any of them.

LESSON LEARNED

You have to take care of yourself. The other doctors, preoccupied with their own agendas, may not watch out for you.

The above is one story. Here is another that, to me, is even more chilling. It is told by an intern in another urban hospital.

I got stuck doing a routine blood draw using a butterfly needle. I do so many of them. That was probably my eighth draw of the day. The patient was on the HIV service and admitted with an opportunistic infection. I had drawn his blood before without incident. This time the needle just

21

slipped through my hands as I was taking it out and it punctured my skin. I couldn't believe it. It all happened so fast and I hadn't done anything out of the ordinary. It just slipped. I had heard that others had occasionally been stuck, but I didn't think it would ever happen to me.

I went immediately to the chief resident. I thought he would make a big stink out of it. I thought he would rush me to occupational health and somehow everyone would care—or at least think it was a big deal. This was HIV infected blood. I could feel the heat in my cheeks. I knew my face was red, and I just hoped that I could keep the tears from coming.

"I got stuck while I was drawing patient X's blood."

The chief barely looked up from his chart. "Okay. You can go to occupational health. Just finish your notes and then sign out to Chang."

I didn't know what to do. I waited for a moment, pausing. The chief must not have heard me, and any minute mountains would move and lightning would crash down on the very floor upon which I stood. Didn't anyone realize that I might have just contracted a deadly infection? Time was running out, and no one seemed to think anything had happened. If I didn't start antiretroviral therapy STAT, wouldn't the virus invade and spread through my body? "Don't I need to go now?" I asked.

The chief reluctantly picked his head up out of the chart. "Look, it's no big deal. Get used to it. We all get stuck. If you go to occ health they'll tell you that the risk of transmission of HIV is less than 1%, more like 0.3 or 0.4%. You can take antiretrovirals, which lower your chance of transmission by close to 80%. But if you take them, there are all sorts of nasty side effects."

I stared, stunned by his casualness.

The chief saw the expression on my face and shook his head like he was saying, "Don't you know anything?" "Look," he said to me, "Take Kramer—she got stuck last year and didn't take anything. She was fine. Bryant got stuck last year, too. He took the antiretrovirals for four weeks and spent half that time with flu symptoms, fevers, chills, nausea, vomiting. He was a mess. Sandra got stuck last year, too. She took the antiretrovirals and got a kidney stone. A couple of other people I know have taken the antiretrovirals and have done just fine with them. The bottom line is that there is no good answer. Just pick one. But first finish your notes and then sign out to Chang."

His voice was cold, matter-of-fact, and I think that's what sticks with me most. He was saying: "This is just the way it is, so get used to it." I couldn't accept it at first. But, as time passed and I saw other people get stuck and go through the same thing I did, I realized he was right. This was the cold, awful truth of internship at my hospital. It was dangerous, pure and simple.

LESSON LEARNED

With few exceptions, at no time in your career will you likely be at greater risk of a needle stick than during your internship year. *Every single time* you draw blood, place an IV, or expose yourself to a needle, remember to pause and consider the seriousness of what you are doing. It could be life and death. The moment you are tired and get just a little sloppy could be the moment that forever changes your life. Remember that, and please be careful around needles at all times.

BE SUPERVISED DURING BREAST EXAMS

This nightmare could happen to anyone; it's more of a problem for us guys, but women should be aware as well. As an intern, if you are male and doing a breast or pelvic exam, you should always be supervised by a female. The supervising person can be a resident, nurse, or nursing assistant. Just be supervised. You may feel silly or self-conscious getting supervision, but this "discomfort" on your part is far better than your potential future discomfort if you are later accused of sexual misconduct. Consider the following story, told by one of the interns working in the hospital at the time.

He was a foreign medical graduate and was a little shy but very hard working. We were in a busy, urban hospital and ran the clinic. We were supposed to do a full physical exam, but few people ever did. This foreign graduate had been used to doing everything by the book though, so he did screening breast exams on the female patients. His English wasn't very good, and one of the patients thought that his touching was inappropriate. In all likelihood, the patient had never had a manual breast exam before, because they were not usually done in clinic. She filed a criminal complaint.

The hospital didn't stand behind the intern, and he was promptly fired. He didn't have enough money to pay for his legal defense. The residents and staff took up a collection and paid for an attorney. While awaiting trial, he was denied bail and had to stay in jail. Ultimately, he was found not guilty of the charges. He was released but didn't have enough money for the airplane ride home to his wife and daughter. The residents again took up a collection to help pay for his return trip. We all felt terrible for him.

LESSON LEARNED

The foreign graduate in the above example was a perfect setup for this problem. He didn't speak English well. He was working in a busy clinic where people had come to expect only cursory physical exams. And, he was unsupervised while doing a breast exam (which he rightly thought was his duty to perform). While the foreign graduate had a perfect setup for the miscommunication, it could happen to *anyone unsupervised*. For the above young doctor, the consequences were obviously life changing.

When you see patients, you don't know what is in their heads. The middle-aged woman who seems completely reasonable and comfortable with you may be just that, or she may have a borderline personality, or she may have been molested as a child and be terrified of you touching her but has learned to cover up her fears by being polite, or she may be a con artist down on her luck and looking for a lawsuit to turn her fortune around. The bottom line is you don't know; so don't take the chance. It's simply not worth it.

When you have your own private practice and your own patients, you may decide that you are comfortable with certain patients and less comfortable with others. If your practice involves touching sensitive areas, you may choose to be supervised with all, some, or none of your patients. Fine, that's later. For now, while you're an intern, I would strongly suggest that you be supervised during breast and pelvic exams. Misunderstandings happen all the time. Don't risk it. Your patients won't mind having someone else of the same gender in the room. On the contrary, even if they don't think it is necessary, they will likely appreciate your sensitivity.

25

ADDRESS YOUR PATIENT'S PAIN NEEDS

Pain doesn't kill, but it does debilitate. It does cause suffering, perhaps more than other, more deadly problems such as infections and atherosclerosis. As part of caring for your patient, remember to ask about his or her pain needs. There will be times when you may consciously not give pain medications because you need the pain to guide your exam. This may happen in the emergency room, for example, in a patient with possible appendicitis. But the duration of withholding pain medications should be short. Also, I strongly encourage you to explain to your patient the reason for this withholding. If patients understand why they must endure the pain and that it is expected to be temporary, they will probably be able to endure it with less suffering. Fortunately, pain is now considered one of the five vital signs. More and more, pain will be addressed with as much attention as a patient's temperature. Get used to asking patients if they have any pain and then doing something about it if they do. The following is a chilling example of what can happen when pain needs are ignored. It took place in a large, university-based urban hospital.

> I was doing my usual morning rounds. I came to Ms. R's room. Ms. R was an 86-year-old woman recovering from a knee replacement that was complicated by a stroke. She was kind and courteous. When she saw me come into the room, she burst into tears.
>
> "What's wrong?" I asked. Ms. R had been through a lot but I had never seen her cry.
>
> "Oh, I've been lying here all night. My knee is hurting me so much. I haven't slept a wink."

"Did you ask your nurse for pain medication?"

Of course she had, she told me. She had called the nurse, but the nurse told her that the Percocet prescription I had written had expired. She called the on-call intern who wrote for the Percocet. But, this time Ms. R's pain was worse, and she needed more medication. Ms. R called the nurse again, who called the intern. The intern told the nurse that Percocet was sufficient, and he wouldn't write for anything else. The nurse told Ms. R. When Ms. R protested that she was still in a lot of pain, the nurse took her call bell and placed it out of Ms. R's reach. "Just get some sleep," the nurse told her. "You'll be fine."

"I didn't want to be a problem. I know how busy everyone is. My knee just hurts so much."

I felt terrible. I could see how much discomfort she was in. When I went back to the chart, I saw that she had been taking her Percocet around the clock, every four hours. Clearly, even that had not been enough. I had not meant to neglect her pain, but obviously I had. I had never even asked her about pain. I had just given her Percocet PRN because of the history of knee replacement.

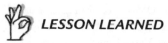 **LESSON LEARNED**

Many patients may feel guilty asking for pain medications. They may not want to appear "weak" or "needy." By nature, they may just be stoic people. They may be afraid that you think they are "drug seeking." Remember to ask your patients about their pain, and address it appropriately. Also, pain prescriptions may need to be refilled, so make sure they don't run out. Don't expect the on-call intern to treat your patient's pain. It's your responsibility. Check whether your patient is actually taking the prescribed pain medication. If the patient is taking the maximum allowed dose every time he or she is allowed to, you may want to consider giving a longer-acting pain medication and then giving a PRN dose for breakthrough pain. Of course, if you *are* the on-call intern and you get a call about a patient's pain, please be sure to address it appropriately, *not* as the intern in the above story did.

ADDRESS DVT PROPHYLAXIS

As soon as a person comes into the hospital as a patient, that person is immediately at risk for a deep vein thrombosis (DVT). Of course, a DVT can lead to a pulmonary embolism (PE), and that can lead quickly to death.

Not every patient you admit to the hospital should receive DVT prophylaxis. There are contraindications to prophylaxis that you need to consider, including, but not limited to, recent hemorrhagic stroke, GI bleed, and/or a clotting factor deficiency. Whether or not a candidate for prophylaxis, every one of your patients should have his or her DVT prophylaxis needs addressed. If not a candidate for anticoagulation, the patient may still benefit from Venodynes.

The trouble is that DVT prophylaxis is all too often overlooked. The patient comes in with pneumonia and so is given antibiotics. Or, the patient has a heart attack and undergoes a cath or is medically managed. But don't forget to address the patient's needs for DVT prophylaxis. Consider the following incident that occurred at a large community hospital.

Our patient was doing well. She was recovering from a glioblastoma resection. Her prognosis was poor given her tumor, but she was up and walking and feeling better. Her family visited every day and, all things considered, she seemed in good spirits. She had some mild leg swelling in the morning and so I ordered a Doppler to rule out a DVT, but my suspicion was low, especially because there was no calf tenderness. She was looking forward to going home in a few days. When I heard the announcement of a code blue in the therapy gym, I was not prepared to find my patient there unresponsive. She had been doing so well. We resuscitated her and got her to the ICU. She stabilized. A CT angiogram was performed and showed a massive saddle PE. The Doppler results also came back and revealed a DVT. I found out the next morning that she had died overnight. It was the worst morning of my internship.

LESSON LEARNED

Some patients are at higher risk for clots than others. Patients with cancer, for example, are at increased risk. Remember to factor in the increased risk, but still always consider and address DVT prophylaxis needs in all your patients. Simply being immobilized in the hospital increases a patient's risk. The above story also underscores an additional important point. Even if your clinical suspicion for a DVT is low, but high enough that you order a Doppler, then you should also order non-weight-bearing status for the involved extremity. Weight bearing on an extremity with a DVT might facilitate dislodging of the clot. If you think it might be there, make the patient non-weight-bearing and rule out the clot. Having said all that, don't lose the forest for the trees. If a patient is septic, your first

29

priority is to control the infection. But, at the same time, remember to address DVT prophylaxis.

REMEMBER TO ADD A BOWEL REGIMEN

Constipation is less dramatic and doesn't have a mortality rate associated with it—but to the patient, I assure you, it is a very serious complication. If you leave constipation untreated for too long and it progresses, then your patient may need disimpaction. Besides the great disregard to the patient by allowing him or her to lie in so much discomfort, guess who gets to do the disimpaction? It's almost certainly not going to be your attending or resident.

As an intern, you can remind your team to be sure to consider adding a bowel regimen. Your team will thank you for thinking of it and appreciate that you are thinking of your patient's well-being. The following incident occurred in a small community hospital.

It was my fourth month of internship. I thought I was finally getting the hang of things. We were treating Mr. J for pneumonia with IV antibiotics. He seemed like an uncomplicated case when he began to develop stomach pain. When I questioned him, I found out that he hadn't had a bowel movement in more than a week. "Not since a day before coming to the hospital, doc," he told me.

I had written for Colace and senna PRN, but he had never asked for them. For my part, I had never asked him if he was moving his bowels.

I started him on an aggressive bowel regimen, including enemas and suppositories, but we were already too far behind the game. We couldn't get him to go. The attending told my resident to digitally disimpact him. My resident told me to digitally disimpact him. I wrote an order for the nurse to digitally disimpact him. The nurse paged me and informed me that nurses didn't digitally disimpact patients at our hospital. Doctors did. So, I gloved up and went in. In the end, Mr. J thanked me. But neither of us enjoyed the procedure.

LESSON LEARNED

Make it a habit to ask your patients if they are moving their bowels on admission and then every day while they are in the hospital. Order bowel regimens if appropriate. If your patient is constipated and not taking PRN bowel meds, consider changing the patient to standing doses to make sure the patient gets them. Do write holding parameters for stool softeners and pro-motility agents (e.g. "Hold for loose bowel movements"). It is a lot easier to manage a patient's bowels *before* they get significantly constipated than it is afterward. Of course, there are other contraindications to a bowel regimen such as GI infection. Regardless of whether or not you end up giving the bowel regimen, you will help ensure that you are being a thorough physician by considering it.

STAY AWAKE IN THE OR BUT SPEAK UP IF YOU CAN'T

The following incident, which took place in a small, wealthy community hospital, is more of a problem in the operating room, but the moral is applicable to any rotation.

Emily was retracting for her fifth straight hour. It was a long surgery and she couldn't even see what was going on. She was told to keep retracting. You know how it is. Anyway, she started to get faint and wobbled a little. The last thing she said she remembered was the surgeon telling her to be still. Then she hit the ground and smashed her head. No one caught her because they didn't want to violate sterile conditions! Emily was taken to get a head CT, which, fortunately, was normal.

LESSON LEARNED

Clearly, the surgeon, other residents, and staff in the OR had some responsibility for Emily falling to the ground and nearly cracking her head open. But Emily bears some of the blame, too. If you are about to pass out, speak up! If you can't hold your bladder anymore, speak up! I'm sure Emily felt intimidated and just wanted to do a good job. My heart goes out to her, and I can't understand the mentality of a surgeon who doesn't care that his intern is standing still for five hours, not even able to see the operating field, without a break. I also can't understand why none of the other people in the room, seeing that Emily was about to fall (as they reported later they did), tried to help her.

Give her a hand, a knee, something to keep her from smashing her skull onto the hard floor! But, a lesson to learn is that you can't change other people. Emily can't make other people on her surgical team care about her or what she is going through. All she can do is change the way *she* acts and reacts under the circumstances. That means speaking up sooner and making your voice heard.

Of course you want to be tough, and you don't want to be a "complainer." But you must look after your own needs. People may be irritated in the short run, but I have to believe they will respect you for it in the long run.

In a self-defense class, I heard an instructor tell his trainees that, if attacked, they should protect themselves as if they were protecting their children. A woman with a young child will no doubt fight bitterly to the end to protect her child. Yet for some reason, when that same woman is alone, the instructor said, she seems less likely to fight as hard for herself. She seems more likely to be conciliatory and try to reason her way out of the situation with the evil attacker. Instead, this self-defense instructor urged his class to take as good care of themselves as they would their children. Similarly, I would ask you to believe that you are entitled to be treated as well as you would want your son or daughter treated. Or, put it this way: Demand to be treated with as much respect as you would treat your intern when you are an attending. Of course, as you do this demanding, be respectful. But, don't think that you can't be respectful and speak up for yourself at the same time.

ORDER LABS FOR THE RIGHT REASONS

One of the tricky parts of being an intern is that you will have different attendings and residents who treat patients, well, differently. Some attendings want labs every day, some only want those that they feel will change the course of treatment.

If a patient falls and bumps her head, some physicians will immediately get a head CT to rule out a bleed. They'll say, "You have to cover yourself, doctor. What if she has a bleed? We can't afford to miss that. Sure, she looks fine and she probably is. But what if she isn't? If she were your mother, wouldn't you want the CT ordered? It's only money. Get the head CT."

For the exact same patient, other physicians will say, "The patient looks fine, let's hold off on the head CT. I want neuro checks q2 hours. If you notice any changes on her exam, then get the head CT. If not, let's hold off. After all, we can't just order head CTs on every patient who falls and has a little bump on the head, can we? Who is going to pay for all those head CTs? A CT scan is an expensive test. It's irresponsible to order every conceivable test just to make yourself feel better. If she fell at home and bumped her head, would she get a head CT then? And what about the radiation exposure? Practice responsible medicine, doctor. If you order every test that ever comes to your head, you'll be bankrupting the medical care system; then when someone really needs a test, they won't be able to get it. Learn to trust your history and physical exam. Your clinical exam is cheap, and if you're good at it, it's as reliable as—or more reliable than—most expensive tests."

Who is right? Neither and both. The truth is that there is more than one way to do things. Every physician practices medicine in a slightly different manner. As an intern, you'll need to adapt to the physician with whom you happen to be working. But that's a good thing. It gives you the opportunity to see how different docs do things, so you can pick and choose the best from all of them. A common example in the hospital is ordering INRs on patients on Coumadin. I have worked with some physicians who—no matter how stable the INR or how many years the patient has been on the same dose of Coumadin—want that INR checked daily. Other physicians are content to check the INR once or twice a week if the INR is very stable and the patient has a stable dosage. As the intern, you can decide which way you would ultimately like to practice, but you have to practice in the moment according to your attending's rules.

I think it is completely wasteful and cruel to order routine labs on patients when there is no reason or need for them. If they're not going to change treatment and you have no reason to suspect that they will be abnormal, why check them? If the patient were at home, would you be checking daily labs just for the sake of it? In many hospitals, "morning labs" means the patient will be woken around 5 or 6 AM to get stuck with a needle. If you can avoid sticking your patient, I would advise it. Of course, always order any labs that are appropriate.

Now, here is the caveat. If your attending physician wants routine labs every day for no apparent reason other than he or she feels they are important, you can gently argue the point with him, but in the end do what he asks. In the end, it is his patient, and he is running the show. If you argue the point, he may respond, "While the patient is in the hospital, I just want to keep an eye on things. I want to make sure we're not missing anything. When the patient goes home, then we'll stop checking daily labs." I don't agree with this. I don't understand why you should check a metabolic panel every day on a young patient who is admitted for a hip fracture and has no risk factors for other disease. But for now I would advise that you ask your attending why and then do as you were instructed and order the labs.

👍 FOLLOW UP ON LABS

Sometimes labs get ordered and you're not sure why. They weren't your idea, but there they are—ordered. Your resident or attending may have ordered them. Your consultants may have requested that your resident order them or they may have ordered them themselves. The point is that if it's your patient and the labs are ordered, you need to check them.

> *"How was I supposed to know that the patient had a potassium of 6? I didn't even order the metabolic panel."*
>
> *"Isn't this your patient?" asks the attending.*
>
> *"Yes."*
>
> *"Then you need to know the potassium level, don't you?"*
>
> *"Yes, but I didn't order it."*
>
> *"It doesn't matter."*

 LESSON LEARNED

The above situation will happen. It's not fair, but it will happen. Ideally, the person who ordered the labs should let the rest of the team know that he or she ordered them, and that person should also check them. After all, he or she ordered them! But it doesn't always work that way. Attendings will come by and, almost on a whim, decide that checking a CBC, BMP, x-ray, or Doppler is a good idea. They may not even write it in the chart. Or if they do write it, it may be illegible chicken scratch. They should write it and write it legibly, but they might not. Either way, they will still expect you to check on the results. In the worst scenario, the potassium is 7, and no one checks it. The patient has an arrhythmia and dies, and you get blamed for not checking it.

👍 REVIEW YOUR PATIENTS' ACTUAL FILMS AND TESTS

It can be frustrating and a bit tedious at times to stare at films when you don't know what you're looking at. During internship, everyone brings with them a different amount of experience reading films. Some can read plain chest x-rays, some can't. Few feel comfortable reading CT scans or MRIs. Regardless of your previous experience level, internship and residency in general will provide you with ample opportunity to get a firm grasp of the basics. The trouble is that when it's 3:30 PM and you have a list of things to do and want to go home by 5 PM (or close to it), it's tempting to just ask the radiologist for the results rather than actually going to look at the film yourself.

To be certain, the goal of internship is not to become an expert radiologist. The goal is not even to become an adequate radiologist. Radiologists have their own residencies and fellowships. But you certainly can and should learn the basics. Here is why:

Learning the basics of reading films and actually *seeing* the pathologies that you are otherwise trying to diagnose and treat laid out for you on film can really make medicine come alive for you. It can take an abstraction and make it less abstract. You know what a bleed in the head is and what the ramifications might mean, and you trust that the radiologist can read the head CT better than you or your medicine attending can, but somehow *seeing* it on the CT scan can make the clinical points stick better.

There may be times when you want a film read and there is no radiologist available. This could be during residency or perhaps when you are in your own practice. You may order a film and no one is available to read it. Being able to make out the basics in that instance—to distinguish heart failure from pneumonia, for example, can be extremely useful to you and your patient.

Depending on your ultimate field of specialization, you may indeed need or want to become very good at reading certain kinds of films. Learning the basics during internship and residency will greatly help as you refine the skills for your specialty.

Once you agree that it is useful to learn the basics of reading films (and one hopes most of you will), the next logical question is how best to achieve this radiological competence. I would argue that the best way to learn to read films is through repetition. Start by learning the very basics. Ask your senior resident, attending, or friendly radiologist to give you a *systematic* approach to looking at various types of films (e.g., x-ray, CT, MRI). Then, simply use that method on as many films as you have the chance to see. Each time you read a film, use your systematic approach until it becomes second nature to you.

Time is extremely precious during internship. No doubt about that. But it doesn't take *that* much time to go over a film. If you can go over it with a more senior person, terrific. If not, it is still worth going through it by yourself. If you feel lost and don't know exactly what you're looking at, that's okay. Go through it systematically, and try to look at it as though you had to present what you see to your attending. Even though it looks confusing and intimidating, slowly but surely you will start to make sense of the different forms and shades. Then, when you get the chance to do an elective with a radiologist, you will have the chance to crystallize your skills, and your confidence will grow. However, if you don't put in the groundwork of looking at scores and scores of films over the year, you won't get as much out of it when you finally do sit down to "learn" radiology on an elective. No one will necessarily tell you that you *have* to look at the films for yourself. But if you take it upon yourself to invest the time and effort when you're an intern, you'll be grateful when you're a senior resident.

👍 BE AWARE THAT TEST RESULTS AREN'T ALWAYS 100% ACCURATE

In general, vitals are usually correct, x-rays are read correctly, and lab technicians are very good at reporting accurate results. But not always. You have two important defenses against simply trusting reported test results. First, confirm the results yourself. If you don't trust a set of vitals, repeat them yourself. Review films yourself or with your attending when possible.

A patient in the hospital with osteoporosis had hip, leg, and groin pain after a fall. An x-ray was ordered. The report of the x-ray was filed into the computer: Normal study; no fracture. The intern took the patient off bed rest, despite being concerned about the level of pain the patient was still having. The attending didn't believe the x-ray result. She went down with the team and looked at the film herself. There was a clear intertrochanteric fracture. The radiologist, it turned out, hadn't missed the fracture. He had just written the report for the wrong patient into the computer. It's not a common mistake, but it happens.

LESSON LEARNED

The second way to defend against erroneous reports of data is to use common sense. Common sense can help save you from numerous mishaps. Make use of this important skill whenever you can. If everyone on your service on a particular wing all of a sudden has a fever, there are several possible explanations: Maybe a virus is going around. Maybe it's a coincidence. Or, as I have heard and seen happen, maybe the thermometer is broken! Similarly, if all of your patients suddenly have a drop of two points in their blood count, maybe the lab has a problem. Try calling the lab or reordering the tests. Also, talk to your colleagues. If all of the patients on more than one service simultaneously have very low potassium levels, then maybe before replacing the potassium, you should check whether the lab is really sure about those results. You don't want to supplement potassium in patients who might have normal or even high potassium levels! Common sense is a useful tool; use it.

40

ALWAYS ASK A CHILDBEARING-AGE FEMALE PATIENT IF SHE IS PREGNANT *PRIOR* TO GETTING AN X-RAY OR CT SCAN AND ALWAYS CONSIDER GETTING A β-HCG

The following took place in an urban hospital clinic. The intern telling this story was, by all accounts, an excellent and meticulous worker. This just serves to illustrate that these mistakes can happen to anyone.

I saw an overweight 14-year-old girl in the clinic. Her mother had brought her in because the girl had fallen a week earlier and had been walking with a slight limp ever since. The girl said she had some groin pain. I did an exam and she didn't have any pain with internal or external rotation of her hip. There wasn't any tenderness. I remembered that in someone her age I had to worry about things like slipped capital femoral epiphysis (SCFE) and Legg-Calvé-Perthes disease, which could be hard to pick up on exam. I ordered x-rays just to make sure everything was intact. I ordered bilateral hip films for comparison and an AP pelvis. I presented the patient to my attending, but the clinic was busy and it was toward the end of the year so the attendings pretty much just let us do what we wanted in the clinic. The patient went for the x-rays, and I told her and her mother to follow up in two weeks.

The next day, the on-call resident paged me. "You're in deep trouble," he told me when I returned the page.

"What happened?" I asked. I was on our one elective for the year so I didn't have any floor patients and couldn't imagine what the problem was.

"That girl you saw yesterday, the one in the clinic who got the hip and pelvis x-rays . . ."

"Yes?"

The on-call resident paused, seeming to try to decide how to tell me. "You have to see it for yourself. Do you have a computer? Can you bring it up on the screen?"

I asked for the MRN (medical record number) and the on-call resident waited on the phone with me as I brought up the images. I wasn't great at reading hip or pelvis x-rays, but this was impossible to miss. On the pelvic x-ray was a clearly defined, undeniable outline of a fetal skeleton. "Mother of . . ." My voice trailed off.

"Yep. The radiologist says she's in her second trimester."

I cringed.

"Nice screw up," he told me as if he were saying, "Boy, am I glad that I'm not you right now."

My attending was not as upset as I had expected. I called the patient and told her. We gave her a referral to the obstetrics clinic. I called the clinic myself to arrange the appointment. That was the last I heard of her, but I often think of her and hope I didn't harm her unborn baby.

LESSON LEARNED

The moral here is clear. If you are going to order an x-ray or CT on any female patient of childbearing age, always ask if there is a possibility of her being pregnant and always consider getting a β-HCG. If the answer is yes, just get the β-HCG. If she says no, but you have your doubts, tell her you need to test her anyway. If you're in the ER, get the β-HCG as a screening test regardless. Likewise, before giving any medications to a female of childbearing age, find out if she might be, or is thinking about becoming, pregnant. Depending on the answer you receive, and your relationship with the patient, you still might give the medication or get the test, but at least you can help your patient make an informed decision. The last thing you want is to injure your patient or your patient's unborn baby.

👍 REMEMBER TO CALCULATE THE CORRECTED CALCIUM LEVEL

You've learned it. I know you have. You know you have. So why do so many interns forget to check the corrected calcium level? To remind you, as a general rule, if the calcium level is abnormal, make sure you have checked the albumin level before jumping to any conclusions. Similarly, if for any reason you are concerned about the calcium level, and the calcium comes back normal, make sure you know what the albumin level is before assuming everything is fine. I have not heard of any serious problems resulting from a mistake of calcium calculation, but it wouldn't surprise me. Often, a resident or attending catches the mistake (if one has been made). The more common experience that I have seen many times looks like this:

"And how were Mr. Z's labs?"

"His potassium is a little low, I gave him some K-Dur. Everything else is fine."

"How low?"

"3."

"How much K-Dur?"

"20 milliequivalents."

"Okay, give that times three, Matt," responded the senior resident, rubbing her eyes. "Let's go to rounds."

Later, while walking through rounds, they came back to Mr. Z. The attending, an older male doctor with a jutting

43

forehead, a sloping nose, and large round glasses, asked Matt about his patient.

"He's doing well," Matt responded. "No complaints today. GI is going to see him tomorrow. Until then, we're just waiting."

The glasses slipped down the attending's nose, and he deftly pushed them back on his face. "Labs?" He breathed, almost a sigh.

"Potassium was a little low. We replaced it. Everything else is fine."

"Really?" The attending readjusted his glasses, again. He stood and looked at Matt as if he should say something.

Matt fumbled through his notes. He knew there must be something else there but wasn't sure what. "Well, I guess his calcium was a little high. But not much. It's only 10.7 and upper normal is 10.5. I figured we'll repeat it tomorrow to monitor it."

"Dr. Steffi, did you teach your intern about the importance of a corrected calcium level, especially in a patient such as Mr. Z who is clearly malnourished?"

"Yes, of course." Now the resident's voice was more strident. "Matt, you told me the labs were fine. What is the albumin level?"

"Albumin? I don't know. We didn't check that."

"Dr. Steffi," the attending broke in. He took off his glasses and wiped them, returning them to his face. It seemed the glasses just wouldn't stay put. "Why didn't you check the albumin?"

"I'm sorry," Dr. Steffi responded, "I thought we had. We'll check it stat."

"Is that fair, Dr. Steffi, to give the patient an extra needle stick because you forgot to add a lab? Call the lab and see if they can run it on the blood sample they have before you go sticking Mr. Z again."

For his part, Matt cringed. The harder it got on his resident, the more disagreeable she would be and the harder life would become for him.

✋ LESSON LEARNED

All of this could have been easily avoided. The total amount of calcium varies with the level of albumin in the body, because calcium binds to albumin. The biologic effect of calcium comes from ionized calcium, not total calcium. Ionized calcium does not bind albumin. You can arrive at a corrected calcium level by using a simple formula:

Corrected calcium (mg/dL) = Patient's measured total calcium + 0.8 (4 − patient's serum albumin)

The 4 in the above equation represents an average albumin level. From this formula, you can see that if the albumin level is low, the corrected calcium level (meaning the true amount of calcium) is higher than the total calcium reported from the lab. This calculation works fairly well. One caveat is that it does not work in patients with elevated serum paraproteins (e.g., with multiple myeloma).

Get in the habit of asking yourself what the albumin level is whenever you are getting a calcium level. Attendings and senior residents may not be blown away and start singing your praises if you calculate the corrected calcium level (as they shouldn't), but they'll be impressed that you're thinking, and every once in a while you will save your senior an embarrassing moment, and thus save yourself your senior's post-embarrassing-moment grumpiness.

👍 KNOW HOW TO CLEAN AND PRESERVE AN AMPUTATED FINGER APPROPRIATELY

In some ways, emergency rooms are among the most exciting places for an intern to spend a rotation. The pace is quick, the acuity is greatest, and the volume of work often means that interns have the opportunity to work with the least supervision in the initial patient encounter, workup, and sometimes management. Of course, for all the same reasons, emergency rooms tend to elicit interns' mistakes. Here is one such example. Interestingly, the following incident didn't take place in a busy, urban medical center. Rather, this was in the emergency room of a relatively quiet community hospital in an affluent zip code that was having an unusually busy night. The person telling the story was a resident at the time it occurred.

There must have been a full moon or something because we had several traumas that night. Usually, at most we'd have one or two. Anyway, one of the patients who came to the ER was a guy who had been working in his garage and managed to sever the distal part of his second finger. His wife had frantically driven him to the hospital. Jen was the first to see him. She was a pretty good intern, but this was her first rotation in the ER. Usually an intern wouldn't have seen a traumatic amputation by herself, but, like I said, things were busy that night. The wife gave her the digit in a plastic bag. Jen immediately got a bag of ice and put the digit, still in the plastic bag, into the ice. Then, thinking she had time with the finger on ice, she set about taking a quick history from the patient and examining the bloody stump.

The typical course in the ER was for the intern to examine the patient and order any necessary labs, films, etc. If the intern wasn't sure, then he or she was to grab an attending and present the case immediately. Jen knew enough to know that she wasn't comfortable treating a traumatic digit amputation by herself. She ordered the man some pain medication and went straight to her attending.

"What do you have?" The attending asked.

"Traumatic amputation," Jen replied. "Second digit distal to the proximal interphalangeal joint."

"Does he have the severed digit with him?"

"Yes."

"Good. Can he wait a minute?"

"Yes, he's okay. I gave him some pain meds. He's just scared about what is going to happen to his finger."

"Okay. Call hand and microsurgery and see who is covering. I'll be there in just a minute."

A few minutes later, the attending came to the bedside. His face, already ruddy from overwork and lack of sleep, became redder. He took the amputated digit in the bucket and carried it away. "Come with me," he said to Jen, leaving the patient and his wife.

The attending removed the amputated digit and gently washed it in sterile saline, placing saline dipped gauze around it when he was finished. Then he placed it in a new plastic bag, sealed it, and put the bag in an ice and saline slush. When he was done, he turned to Jen.

"Never put an amputated digit directly on ice, doctor," he told her. "If it freezes, that's the end of your digit. Put it in an ice and saline sludge. Never just ice. And when you irrigate," he continued, "irrigate gently. Let vascular or microsurgery be the ones to do the delicate debriding. If we debride too aggressively, we risk killing vital structures, which would make it hard to reattach the finger."

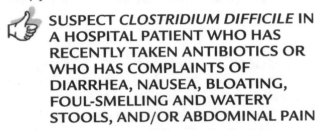

LESSON LEARNED

Jen's mistake is a common one. We are used to hearing that you should put an amputated digit "on ice." After all, that's what they seem to do on television! But, as Jen learned by almost killing a finger, doing this can cause the finger to freeze. It is important to put an amputated body part in cold water and ice, but not directly on ice.

SUSPECT *CLOSTRIDIUM DIFFICILE* IN A HOSPITAL PATIENT WHO HAS RECENTLY TAKEN ANTIBIOTICS OR WHO HAS COMPLAINTS OF DIARRHEA, NAUSEA, BLOATING, FOUL-SMELLING AND WATERY STOOLS, AND/OR ABDOMINAL PAIN

The following occurred in a community hospital.

A nurse was admitted to the hospital for an elective total hip replacement. Post-op, she developed a urinary tract infection. She was treated with antibiotics and was to be discharged but then developed severe abdominal cramping. The nurse had a host of other medical problems and a large workup ensued to identify the source of her abdominal symptoms. It wasn't until she had suffered through about a week of endoscopies and various scans that one of the doctors sent her stool for C. difficile. *The stool tested positive for the toxin. The nurse was promptly started on metronidazole and got better.*

LESSON LEARNED

C. *difficile* infection presents in a variety of ways. It doesn't always have diarrhea or foul smelling stools

48

associated with it. The lesson here is to consider *C. diffi-cile* in any patient who has recently been treated with antibiotics and has abdominal complaints. It is, after all, an easy test to send and something that can be readily treated once diagnosed. Likewise, any patient who is immunocompromised and has abdominal com-plaints, particularly an inpatient in a hospital, should be considered for *C. difficile* infection. That doesn't mean you have to test all of them—but keep it in mind and be ready to raise it to your attending as part of your differential diagnosis.

BORROW BLANKETS FROM THE ER WHILE ON CALL

Some call rooms, as you probably already know, are cold. If your call room is kept cold, bring extra clothes for the night. Also, consider going to the ER to see if they have blankets that you can borrow for the evening. I don't know if all ERs do this, but most ERs that I have worked in have had a stash of warm blankets. I always asked before taking, but no one ever had a problem with a cold medical student or resident borrowing one to help keep warm while on call. Keep this in mind if you're stuck in the call room and it's cold!

MAKE SURE YOUR PATIENT HAS APPROPRIATE FOLLOW-UP CARE ARRANGED UPON DISCHARGE FROM THE HOSPITAL

Unless told otherwise, when you discharge patients home from the inpatient floor and write their outpatient prescriptions, make absolutely certain that he or she has an arranged follow-up care plan as an outpatient. Don't oblige if those patients call you in a month asking for refills.

The following story was related to me by a resident who did her internship in a large university hospital.

I was walking with my friend and she got a page from the operator.

"Yes, this is Dr. Doe . . . Oh, hello Mr. Crane. Yes, I remember. Um, okay. Remind me of the phone number. Wait, hold on. Okay, I have a pen. Go. Yes . . . yes . . . alright, I'll call it in. Has everything been going okay? . . . Good. . . . It's still 25 of the hydrochlorothiazide and the Prevacid, right? Yes . . . okay. . . . You know, I can't keep doing this for you. . . . I know. . . . I know. . . . Okay, no problem. . . . You, too, bye."

"What was that?" I asked her as we headed for the cafeteria.

"Oh, he's a patient I had a few rotations ago. Mr. Crane. We discharged him, and I can't get him to follow up with his doctor, so I keep refilling his prescriptions. He says he is look-ing for a new doctor since they moved apartments. Anyway, it's just HCTZ and Prevacid, but it's a royal pain. I have to call the pharmacy. Hold on."

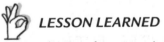 *LESSON LEARNED*

Depending on how your inpatient service is run, you may be called upon to write prescriptions that patients fill at their local pharmacy after discharge. At my intern-ship, for whatever reasons, the residents always did this. But, I know of many other internship programs in which the interns had this responsibility. When the medication runs out, assuming it is a medicine that the patient is supposed to be on for more than the duration of the prescription given, the patient may call *you* for a refill. As a resident, I was paged on several occasions by patients asking me for a refill of medicine. There are two important reasons *not* to do this.

First, you are not the patient's primary care doctor. You don't know what has been going on since you last saw the patient in the hospital. If you refill a prescription, thinking that it is okay for him or her to continue on the medicine, it may be okay or it may not. Maybe something has changed. Maybe the patient wants a refill of atorvastatin, but unbeknownst to you, the patient's liver enzymes are rising and no one is checking. If you give the patient a refill, you are legally saying that you are still caring for the patient. If something goes wrong, *you* are responsible. You don't know what medications the patient may now be taking. Maybe he or she does have another doctor and maybe this doctor decided to start giving the patient Coumadin for his or her heart valve. Or maybe the patient has started taking another medication that can also have hepatotoxicity. When the patient calls you, you aren't going to be able to ask all the appropriate questions, and even if you could ask all the questions you would want, you still need to lay eyes on the patient and do an exam (not to mention update the medical record) if you wanted to take the patient as your own—which you don't because you're an intern and aren't ready for your own private practice yet.

Second, even if you thought the patient was asking for a benign medication to refill, and you didn't mind the added risk and liability to yourself, you would still be doing your patient a disservice. Your patient should have an attending physician overseeing his or her care. If he or she is calling you and asking for refills, then the patient doesn't have a primary care physician managing his or her medical needs. If you refill the medications, you are facilitating this lack of appropriate follow-up care, which means the patient is not getting good care. If he or she is getting follow-up care, then *that* doctor should be writing the prescriptions, not you.

There is a simple and effective way to protect yourself against receiving this call. Don't discharge a patient until and unless he or she has adequate and appropriate follow-up care. This is something you and your team should be (and hopefully are) doing anyway. But sometimes it falls through the cracks, especially with service patients who don't have insurance. Don't let it fall through. Make sure there is a doctor who knows about the patient and is prepared to follow up with him or her. The patient should have an appointment with the doctor upon discharge from the hospital and a way of getting to that appointment. Your social worker can be very helpful in this regard.

I also think it is wise to only write for one month of medication when discharging a patient from the hospital. If you write for a month of medicine, and give four refills, you're inviting the patient to not follow up with the doctor until the refills run out. But five months is *too long* for most patients to wait to follow up with their doctors after leaving the hospital. People are people—we all enjoy convenience, and none of us wants or likes to be sick. Many people will avoid the doctor if possible. This is particularly true when a patient goes to the hospital, starts on the right medications, and then feels better and is discharged. It is natural that some people in this situation will want to avoid doctors and hospitals and just continue on the medications that are making them feel better. And, you do them a service if you encourage them to attend their appointment with their doctor after leaving the hospital. One of the ways you encourage them to follow up with their doctor is to make sure they need to see the doctor to get prescription refills. After all, a lot can change in five months, and you want to make sure that the patient is getting the right medications. Especially in these days of intense insurance scrutiny, few people are admitted to the hospital who don't really need to be there. Anyone who needs to be in the hospital requires close follow-up after being discharged. If it's a clinic patient, make sure the patient has an appointment with the appropriate clinic prior to discharge.

If you *are* called for a refill of medication, I would encourage you to explain to such patients that you are not their primary care physician. You were taking care of them while they were in the hospital, but now they need to have their own primary care doctor who, incidentally, you had set them up with prior to leaving the hospital. If they protest or if they say that they had been meaning to go to their doctor but hadn't had a chance to yet, let them know that you would be doing them a disservice to treat them from the hospital, especially as you are not qualified and they require *and deserve* professional care from a physician who actually sees them in their office. Again, do your best to preempt the conversation by arranging for outpatient follow-up. You can even explain to such patients prior to discharge that you will not be continuing with their care and that they must follow up with the physician with whom they have the appointment.

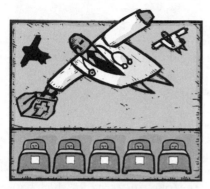

Chapter 3

Rounds: Do's and Don'ts

👍 WAKE UP YOUR PATIENTS IN THE MORNING

Even when you really don't want to and think it's cruel, it's important to make sure your patients are awake in the mornings. If you like to sleep as much as I do, you probably feel as guilty as I used to waking patients up at the crack of dawn. There are a lot of aspects of hospitals that don't make a lot of sense. For example, isn't sleeping a vital component to healing? Is that such a radical thought? Why don't we let patients get a good night's sleep? Is putting an occasional sign up saying, "Patient area, please keep quiet after 8 PM" the best we can do to encourage a good night's sleep? How about *not* drawing their blood at 4 AM? How about not having all of the machines around them and attached to them beep, buzz, and flash? And, how about us doctors *not* waking them up in the morning?

As much as I hated waking up patients in the morning, it was and is a necessary evil until hospital policies or residency policies change. Maybe this is one of the battles you want to pick with your director—but it's not one you are likely to win. In any case, until your attending stops requiring that you know how your patients are doing before morning rounds, wake them up and ask them how they are feeling, even when you would rather not. Consider the following scenario, which happens on a daily basis in hospitals across the country.

"Mr. Jones? Mr. Jones?"

"Yes," a sleepy voice replies.

"I'm sorry to wake you. It's Dr. Intern. Good morning. How are you?"

"What? Oh, hi, Doctor. I'm fine."

"That's good. Do you have any chest pain or shortness of breath?"

"No."

"Are you moving your bowels?"

"What?"

"Bowels. Have you had a bowel movement? 'Poo poo.'"

"Oh, yes, yesterday."

"Good. Did you sleep okay?"

"Not really."

"Okay, I'm just going to listen to your heart and lungs. Breathe in . . . and out . . . good. You can go back to sleep now. Breakfast should be here in about an hour. Try to get a little more rest."

"No, it's okay, I'm up."

"No, go back to sleep. I just wanted to make sure you were okay. I'll see you later."

LESSON LEARNED

I have to believe that someday we won't wake patients early in the morning in hospitals. We'll come to understand and internalize the notion that sleep is a necessary component of healing. Never mind that *we* feel awful when we don't sleep and we're young and healthy. No, one day we'll realize that our patients, with all of their medical problems, also feel terrible when they don't get a good night's sleep—which is most nights in the hospital. Maybe it will take a forward-thinking hospital to fund a small study showing that patients who are given the proper conditions (e.g., quiet, darkness, better-timed blood draws) sleep better and get better sooner, costing less money to the insurance companies. Once that study gets out, insurance companies will, one hopes, offer incentives to hospitals to encourage good sleep hygiene and then, and most likely only then, will we see real change. Until that day, wake your patients. If you fail to do this, the following story, which happened to an unlucky intern in an urban hospital, could be you.

My attending asked me how Mrs. X was doing and if she still had any pain. I told him Mrs. X was doing well, no complaints, no pain. Mrs. X was a nice, elderly lady in the hospital with a second MI. My attending always asked if she was still having pain, but she hadn't had pain since her admission. She was improving and getting ready for discharge. I had rounded on her that morning. Her vitals were stable, and nothing had happened overnight. I went in to see her, but she was sleeping so soundly. I was in a hurry anyway, so I let her sleep.

We went up to Mrs. X's room. She was still in bed. Her breakfast was in front of her but she hadn't touched it.

"Good morning, Mrs. X," my attending said. "Mrs. X?"

Mrs. X opened her eyes and smiled, but something wasn't right. She wasn't her usual self. "Uh oh," I thought. "Mrs. X?" I said, moving past my attending and shaking her arm.

Mrs. X kept opening her mouth like she was trying to talk, but nothing came out. My attending said, "Zach, this must have happened in the last hour since you saw her."

Trapped, I responded: "Well, she was sleeping before. I didn't really wake her that much. She seemed okay."

"I'm confused. How did you know she didn't have any pain? You did or did not talk to her?"

"I did not. I just eyeballed her. I'm sorry."

LESSON LEARNED

The intern in the above story felt awful but did not get into trouble. Still, his not wanting to wake Mrs. X in the morning was a big mistake. If he had woken her, maybe they would have found out she was having a stroke earlier, and maybe they could have helped her more. Probably not, since it was ischemic and not a bleed, and she was not a candidate for thrombolytic treatment. Still, he should have known. And, if he had woken her earlier, he would not have been caught lying to his attending. There is little that an attending wants more than an intern who tells the truth, and little less that he or she will tolerate than an intern who does not. So, do your job. Part of your job, unfortunately, until that research study by the forward-thinking hospital is done and the rules are changed, is to wake your patient early in the morning.

Although in the above scenario, Mrs. X might have been helped by being woken earlier, this example does

58

not argue for waking all patients early every morning. The story of Mrs. X was a chance occurrence that could have happened at *any* time. In Zach's case, he was instructed to see her; he *said* he had done so, but hadn't. He should have. However, to use the above incident as an excuse to argue for waking all patients up early would also suggest the following: We should wake patients every hour during the night just to check that they are not having a stroke or other event. Of course, that is a ridiculous notion.

REPORT ACCURATE, HONEST INFORMATION ON ROUNDS

This is a big one and probably one of the most practical pieces of advice that you should institute on a daily basis. Of course you know not to make up information on rounds or anywhere else. You don't need to be told this. And yet, there are innumerable examples I could give for this one. I've seen it happen almost every year of medical school and residency. Here is a benign example, representing a common occurrence:

You are an intern going on rounds with your team. The attending asks you about patient X's potassium level. The potassium? You have twelve patients on your service, you're post-call, you have slept only minutes in the past 24 hours, you just started your internship, three of your patients are really sick, and this attending—who, by the way, looks very well-rested, well-groomed, and unhurried—is asking you about the potassium of one of your few healthy patients? Who cares? It was normal; isn't that enough? You know he wants an exact value, and if you don't know it, he'll say, "Why don't

59

you know the potassium level? Isn't patient X your patient? Aren't you taking care of him?" So you say, "4.6." After all, you're sure it was close to that, and normal is normal. Why should you get in trouble for not knowing the exact number?

LESSON LEARNED

Nine times out of ten in the above example, if you behaved as described, you'd be fine. The attending would nod and move on to the next question. But what about that tenth time? He would call you on it and say, "No, it was 4.2." I've seen it happen countless times, especially with new interns whom the attendings are testing. Attending physicians know what it is like to start a new internship. Once upon a time, however hard to believe, they were there. They know you can't know everything, and they know when they're asking a small detail that they don't expect you to have at your fingertips. The correct way to handle the above scenario is to say something like, *"It was normal. I'm not sure of the exact value but I can check if you'd like."* There—now you're covered. Sometimes attendings are just testing you to make sure they can trust you. If they find that they can't, your life quickly becomes much more difficult. Sometimes, attendings simply want to assert their authority and keep you on your toes by asking for details they know you probably don't know. Whatever their motivation, always tell the truth. Consider the following less benign example.

The attending asks you if the routine labs were normal on a given patient. You forgot to check them, but you figured they were probably normal. After all, they had been normal for the last week. So you say that, yes, they were normal. You tell yourself that you're not jeopardizing patient care because you'll check later to make sure. But, then rounds end and you go on to the hundred other things you have to do and you forget again about the labs. So they don't get checked. Of course, in the worst case of the above example, the patient has an electrolyte imbalance (maybe he's on Lasix or something else or maybe he's just unlucky), and he has an arrhythmia and dies.

LESSON LEARNED

This is certainly a rare occurrence, and I've never witnessed it or heard about it, but it *could* happen so why take the risk? It's not fair to your patient, and it exposes you to a serious problem. I have seen residents of all levels make this mistake who have had to deal with smaller complications such as missed infections and more benign arrhythmias. If you forgot to check something and someone asks you, just say so. If you don't, you'll regret it at some point. More importantly, one of your patients may end up suffering as a result of your pride, and that is simply not an option.

ALWAYS MAKE SURE YOUR PATIENT IS STABLE EVEN WHEN THE VITALS ARE STABLE

The following happened to a very good friend of mine. He was interning at a busy urban hospital. To be fair, the nurses were overworked and underappreciated. Still, it is hard to fathom the events that unfolded.

My friend came in early to round on his patients. It was about 6:30 AM. Now, everyone had a slightly different routine. My friend's routine was to first check all the vital signs. All of his patients had stable vitals. When he went in to see his second patient of the morning, the patient was dead. Not only that, the patient was cold and stiff. Clearly, he had been dead for hours. There was simply no way this dead man had had a temperature of 36.5 °C, a pulse of 70, respirations of 20, and he certainly did not have a blood pressure of 136/80, yet that was what had been documented in the chart for that patient that morning! In fact, the patient had had normal vital signs throughout the night. But the story gets worse, much worse.

My friend went outside to get his resident, unsure of what to do. The resident came into the room and said, "Well, we have to code him." It was hospital policy to run a code on anyone in the hospital whose heart had stopped beating and who did not have a DNR order. So, they called a code. The code team came and my friend had to start chest compressions on this dead, cold, stiff corpse. Paddles were brought out, and the patient was shocked. They coded the patient for a few minutes and then pronounced him dead. But, wait, the story is not over. Sadly, it gets still worse.

The code team cleared out of the room and left the nurses to clean up. My friend went to the nurse's station to write his note of what had happened. He looked up and saw the nurse come out of the room. As she did, the patient's family was coming around the corner. My friend heard the patient's wife ask where her husband was. The nurse, incredibly, pointed to the room. Pointed to the room! No word about the code or the death. Nothing. Just pointed to the room.

My friend saw it all happening but couldn't believe it. He said by the time he stood up to try to stop them, the wife and her three children were in the room. The next thing he heard was the wife's screams. One of the sons ran out to the nursing station and called for a doctor.

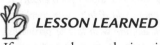 *LESSON LEARNED*

If you spend enough time in the hospital, you will see some wonderful things: acts of kindness and generosity that surpass all expectations. You will see heroism and moments of the most private vulnerability. Unfortunately, you will also see terrible, tragic acts of thoughtlessness. My friend says he can still hear the wife's screams.

In any case, the moral of this lesson is to not assume that just because the vitals are stable, the patient is stable. In this instance, clearly the vitals had been fabricated. But, in general, even if the vitals are real, the patient may be in some distress. Always check on your patients in the morning to make sure they are doing okay. And, if your patient appears to have gotten worse or looks febrile, but the vitals are stable, have the nurse repeat the vitals or, preferably, repeat them yourself.

ALWAYS CHECK VITALS BEFORE REPORTING THEM

This is similar to not making up labs or other information during rounds. But, this one, too, is often violated. Even when a patient's vital signs have been fine for days on end, check them again on each round. Here is the scenario and, unfortunately, it's a common one:

You're running late. One of your patients held you up, and now you're behind. Or maybe you just overslept or were moving more slowly than usual. Whatever the reason, you had to go to rounds with your attending, and you didn't get a chance to see Ms. Jones on the tenth floor. You didn't even check her vitals yet. She is a pretty sick woman with lots of problems, but she has been stable for the past three days. In fact, you are really just waiting for a bed to open up for her at a nursing home before you discharge her. Your attending asks you, "How is everyone?"

Mr. Smith had some shortness of breath, you tell your attending. His lungs were wet so you gave him Lasix. Ms. Brown has abdominal pain. GI wants to get a CT scan. And so on. When you finish your list, or almost finish, your attending says, "Good job." Good job! A rare compliment from your attending. He is finally starting to appreciate your hard work. "Oh," he asks, looking through his list as you start walking to the first patient, "How is Ms. Jones doing today?"

Stop. Before you think about how you would like to answer that question; before you think about how easy it would be to preserve your good favor with your attending and tell him that Ms. Jones is fine just as she has been for the last three days, consider the following incident that took place in a busy urban hospital in New York.

The attending was a real "piece of work." If you missed any detail he would nail you on it. He asked me about patient X, the one patient I hadn't seen yet. I couldn't deal with him drilling or laying into me as usual, so I just told him the patient was fine, had no complaints, and showed stable vitals. I knew the patient was fine. That patient was always "fine," and no one had told me that anything bad happened overnight on sign-out. So, of course the patient was fine. When we got to the floor where patient X was, her cardiologist was at the nursing station with her chart.

"I hear our lady is doing well," my attending said.

I cringed. I knew something was wrong. I could just feel it. The cardiologist, who knew patient X's family well, was never there in the morning.

The cardiologist shook his head. "Didn't you hear? Ms. X died a few hours ago. I had told them to call me if you weren't around so I could tell Mr. X. I've known them for more than twenty years. It's really too bad. I thought she was doing fine."

✌ LESSON LEARNED

No joke. This doesn't happen often, but it happens. Don't make up information about patients. You can be scolded for not having done something in a timely manner—but everyone will understand because they know how busy interns are, and they know how hard you work. Besides, you can always try and be faster next time. But you can be seriously reprimanded and even dismissed for lying. Not to mention that it is bad patient care to lie about their status! There are just no two ways about it. If you make up information— which really means if you lie—you'll eventually get burned. In this case, the intern weathered the storm that came later with the attending and then her program director. But I guarantee you she still wishes that she had just told her attending on that fateful morning that she hadn't yet had a chance to check on Ms. X.

👍 BE SENSITIVE ABOUT CORRECTING YOUR RESIDENT IN FRONT OF YOUR ATTENDING

Your attending will ask questions that your resident won't know the answer to. Sometimes, when your resident doesn't know the answer, you might. What you do with the answer in that situation should depend on three factors. First, what is the culture of your team? Second, what is your direct relationship with the resident and attending? Third, how important is it to you to show that you know something the resident does not?

The culture of your team is very important. When I was a medical student, the surgical residents at one of the hospitals where I rotated told the students, point blank, that if we knew an answer on rounds that they did not, we should keep it to ourselves. Likewise, the senior residents told the same thing to the junior residents, who repeated it in turn to the interns. I never heard such a direct warning when I was an intern, but the implications were there. Know the culture of your team. If you're not sure, you might consider asking, depending on your comfort level.

Your relationship with your resident and attending is also important. Of course, this often reflects on the culture of your team, but not always. I have been on teams of attending and residents where the culture of the entire group is stiff, but the relationship between my resident and me, and the two of us and the attending is more familiar. In that instance, I might feel more comfortable with speaking up. It really depends. But you need to be aware of the dynamics at play.

Only you know how important it is to you that you show that you know something the resident does not.

I would ask you to ask yourself the following question, though: Why is it important to you? Are you unsure of yourself and seeking validation from others? Are you just proud that you know something and want to share it? There is no right or wrong answer to these questions, there is only your truth. And if you know the answers, then you can make informed decisions about how to act.

LESSON LEARNED

Consider the potential negatives to showing up your resident: A pissed-off resident could make your life very difficult. Also, there will be lots and lots of times when your resident will know something that you don't. How do you want the resident to handle those situations? This might be a good moment to start creating some good will so that your resident doesn't make you feel like an imbecile when you don't know something.

Of course, there are also many styles with which you can communicate that you know something. You can declare, "Don't you know, the answer is X." Or, you can say, "I know the answer. It is X." Or, you could be a little more delicate, more political, and say something like, "I think that the answer might be X."

There are stories of interns getting tortured (figuratively, not literally) by their residents after showing the resident up during rounds. You may have stories of your own to this effect. The same dynamic is at play when you are a medical student. However, as an intern, there will likely be more of these instances, particularly as the year progresses. On the whole, residents don't appreciate that. It may be seen as undermining their

67

position. Again, there is no right or wrong in terms of what to do in this situation. Just be aware and be sensitive to it.

TAKE OWNERSHIP OF YOUR PATIENTS' CONDITIONS: TRY TO LEARN EVERYTHING YOU CAN ABOUT THEM

You've heard this before, and, hopefully, you try to already do it. Realistically, though, as an intern (as well as a student), sometimes it can be difficult. As an intern, you won't be expected to know how to manage certain medical issues. Usually, you won't even be asked for an opinion regarding management. If you are asked, it will be to test your critical thinking, rather than because your input is valued. The bottom line is that, depending on the hospital, most of the time you may not be directing the care of your patient. In effect, some interns report feeling more like a glorified secretary to the medical team, rather than one of its doctors.

While you won't be directing the care of your patient, and while you may not always fully understand the reasons behind the care being given to your patient, you will definitely be expected to know everything about your patient. Your attending will expect you to "take ownership" of your patient. In your attending's mind, that means you should know if he had a bowel movement the previous day, if he has special dietary needs, how many days of antibiotics he has had and how many days he still has to go, if labs were ordered and what the results were, if medications were given, and if he has social support at home. When you don't know something, your attending may say something like: "What do you mean you don't know? This is your patient, isn't it, doctor? You need to take ownership of your patient."

It can be frustrating to "take ownership of your patient" when you can't direct their care. In many ways, it's like saying this is "your soccer team" when you are the water boy. True, the team needs water. But you aren't on the field, not really, and you aren't managing the players (not really). Still, you are told you need to understand everything about the players, including how much they ate, what their mental and physical state is, and how they are playing.

✋ *LESSON LEARNED*

Despite the frustration, take ownership of your patients and know everything about them. Here's why: For one, it's your job. For another, and more to the point, taking ownership of your patients will make the whole process much, much more fun and rewarding for you. Here is why: You will learn more quickly, and the quicker you learn, the easier everything will become, and the more you will be able to contribute. Furthermore, when you know everything about your patients, you will have less anxiety because you will feel more in control. You won't dread being asked for the potassium level because you will know it.

Once you know what is happening with your patients, you will be better able to start figuring out *why* things are being done. You can interrogate the consultants and ask why they are suggesting replacing one medication for

69

another. All of this serves to make you *think* more. The more you think and the more you understand, the better you will be able to communicate with your patients. Also, the more you understand about your patients, and *why* tests are being ordered, medications given, procedures performed, etc., the easier it will be for you to remember everything about your patients because it will all start to make sense! As you can imagine, the more work you put in to take ownership of your patients early, the sooner everything gets easier and more fun for you.

GET OVER THE STEEPEST PORTION OF THE LEARNING CURVE QUICKLY

Know why all labs are ordered. Know why each medication is being given. Ask lots of questions.

While internship is a year-long learning process, there is a learning curve, and it is steepest at the beginning. At first, you will need to learn the basics. The basics can be daunting, not because they are difficult or intellectually challenging, but because of the amount of information. Essentially, you will need to learn the mechanics of being an intern and the mechanics of the hospital you are in, as well as basic medical care for your patients. The following are three pieces of specific advice that, from my experience and experiences I have heard from others, I can offer to help you get over the steepest portion of the learning curve quickly. The following story came from a community hospital.

On my third day of internship, I had written all of my notes and was rounding on my patients with the senior resident.

70

"Dan, why are you checking this patient's basic metabolic panel?" asked my senior resident.

To be honest, I hadn't even thought about it. I was just trying to remember where the correct slips were to actually order the panel, and I was trying to remember the password they had given me to check the labs. "What?" I asked.

"The metabolic panel. Do you know why we're checking it?"

I would soon learn that I was both blessed and cursed to have a senior resident who demanded that I give 100%. In the end, it was probably a good thing. At the time, I wasn't so sure. "I thought we checked a metabolic panel on all our patients while they were in the hospital," I responded that day. Okay, I wasn't sure, but it seemed reasonable to keep an eye on their labs while they were under our care, just in case.

"No, we don't do that. Think again. Come on, you must know this. Why the metabolic panel?"

I did know, I realized. I knew that I knew. I just couldn't remember. I couldn't remember anything at that moment. As I said, it was my third day, and I was already appreciating how long a year this was going to be. I hadn't left the hospital before 8 PM on the first two days, and I was on call on that day, anxious about what awaited me overnight. I stared blankly at the chart.

"Why is the patient getting K-Dur?" My resident asked.

"To replace his potassium." That seemed logical.

"Is his potassium low?"

"No."

Silence.

I took a slow, deep breath. "Um," I said, rubbing my eyes. Then it hit me like stepping out onto the beach and feeling a familiar ocean breeze. "Oh, he's on Lasix. Lasix is a loop *diuretic that drops your potassium so we give him the potassium in anticipation that this will happen. I would have to go through the chart but probably he has dropped his potassium in the past while on Lasix. We check the metabolic panel primarily to monitor his potassium level."*

✋ LESSON LEARNED

As I mentioned, being an intern isn't rocket science. It's not even neurosurgery. Most medical students already know that furosemide (Lasix) can decrease potassium levels. It's not that Dan didn't know it, either. It was just that, as he said, he was overworked and thinking of other things. I encourage you not to do that. It's easy to stop thinking. Someone will tell you to write for K-Dur, and you just do it. But it's actually a lot easier to remember that he is on K-Dur if you remember that someone on a loop diuretic might show a drop in potassium and might require potassium supplementation. The sooner you make it a point to understand why your patients are having things done to them, the sooner you will find it much easier to remember what is being done to them. So, know why all labs are ordered.

In a similar vein, know why each medication is being given. If you have a heart failure patient, you can remember that he is taking an ACE-inhibitor, diuretic, beta-blocker and other meds—or you can remember that if you have a heart failure patient, they should be taking certain medications. Then, if your patient isn't on those medications, you will know to ask why he is not. Maybe it was an oversight that you can correct or maybe there is a reason you can learn from. Before you can appreciate the nuances, you need to have the basics.

It doesn't take long to understand why each medication is being given, and it feels good once you do know. It helps you feel more in control while in the hospital.

This brings us to my third piece of practical advice to get over the steepest portion of the learning curve. Do ask lots of questions. This is another way of saying that if you don't know what is going on, *ask*. As an intern, your time to not know things, especially basic things, is running out. As a senior resident, there are certain questions that you should already be able to answer. If you start asking them at that point, it is too late. But as an intern, especially in the beginning of the year, you have pretty much carte blanche to ask questions. Why is this patient on oxygen? Why are we checking the platelet level? What does the CT scan show? How do you read this x-ray? You have a lot of room to ask questions.

To paraphrase an old proverb:

He who doesn't know and asks is ignorant for a moment; he who doesn't ask is ignorant forever.

Don't ask indiscriminately, and don't ask at inappropriate times. If your question is something you know you should know and could look up, just look it up. Don't waste other people's time. It is the real world and you do have to be sensitive to how you are being perceived. But, at the same time, your first priority has to be making sure that you understand what is going on. Think of it this way, if you bury your head in the sand, your patients now and in the future will pay the price. That's not fair to them, and it's not fair to you. You're in training and you're not supposed to know everything—so speak up and ask.

👍 TRY THIS LITTLE TRICK TO MAKE PRESENTING AT ROUNDS AND CONFERENCES MORE FUN

When I was a medical student doing my third-year internal medicine rotation, the intern on my team was an enthusiastic and very competent man named Andy. Of all the things I learned from him, one of the most useful was what he said to me just prior to his medicine morning report presentation.

At morning report in this hospital, many attendings would often show up, so it was a bit more formal than some of the other hospitals where I had worked. Andy was presenting a case that he had seen while on call the previous night. I had not had the same call schedule as Andy that week and so I did not know the patient. At that hospital, call was only until 10 PM, and then night float came on. So it wasn't unusual for us to be awake during the post-call day, but Andy looked particularly bright that morning.

"It's going to be a good case," Andy told me as he went to put his films on the viewing box.

"What is it?" I asked, sipping my morning coffee.

Andy shook his head. "I can't tell you. That would take the fun out of it. You have to figure it out from my presentation."

It struck me then. Most interns, even when they had gotten sleep, looked stressed and nervous prior to presenting at those morning reports. It could be an intimidating situation with so many attendings asking questions. But Andy didn't look stressed. He seemed amused, and I realized why. To Andy, his presentation that morning was a game.

Andy knew what his patient had, but he was the only one (except, of course, his resident). Andy knew the answer, and he would give out the clues that could lead the astute listener to the answer as well. It was up to Andy how he wanted to reveal those clues, and that was part of the game. The result was that while most interns I saw presenting were obviously flustered, trying to remember if there were rales in the right or left lung field, or if the CBC was normal or abnormal, Andy was cool and collected. While other interns felt as though the power lay in the audience, and they were at the audience's mercy, Andy saw it as just the opposite. He had the power, the information. And, it showed during his presentation.

Andy presented with great composure and seemed to genuinely enjoy himself as he saw the audience slowly arrive at the correct diagnosis. It wasn't that Andy knew all the answers to the attendings' questions—he didn't. He knew about as much as the rest of the interns. But when he was asked a question that he couldn't answer, he either looked down at his notes and found the answer, told the audience he and his resident hadn't checked what they were asking, or said, "I don't know." If appropriate, he apologized for the oversight, but he did so without too much fuss. He knew the world wouldn't fall apart if he and his resident hadn't checked something on exam. He didn't flinch or hesitate. He took the lessons that he received from his seniors in the audience and continued with his case. Because of his approach, he and his audience enjoyed his presentation much more than usual.

LESSON LEARNED

I have since tried to often remember that approach whenever I am presenting a case at ground rounds or a conference. I have found this approach to be extremely useful. It both allows me to have more fun, and I think it is more entertaining and interesting for my audience.

I hope it will be helpful for you as well. The point is to think of the process as a game. Remember when you were a child and you played games like 20 questions? Well, it's not all that different. You give clues, and your audience can ask questions if they like. If you think of it this way, you can watch their minds work as they get closer and closer to solving the puzzle. By enjoying it, you will also be more relaxed, and you will come to find that you understand the case that much better. When you know that you understand it, you are less likely to forget pieces of it, and you are also less likely to be rattled if you are asked a question whose answer may not be at the tip of your tongue. If you don't like presenting, or even if you do, I would encourage you to give this approach a try.

BE ON TIME FOR ROUNDS

You already know this. This is an easy one, so why do so many people screw it up? I can't figure it out. Things come up from time to time, and you'll have to be late. But, being late has to be the exception, not the rule. Attendings are busier than you, or at least they think they are. And even if they don't think they're busier, most will not care about your schedule. They expect you to be on time to meet with them. When you're late, they will be upset. When they're upset, your life will be more difficult. It's not that you don't know to be on time; it's just that enough people aren't that it seems to deserve some emphasis.

I had a rotation in which I could always gauge how my next day would go by how well the Yankees performed the night before. My attending was a huge Yankee fan, so if they won, my day would be that much more pleasant. If they lost, my colleagues and I braced ourselves for the day.

LESSON LEARNED

The moral here is that, like it or not, fair or not, your day is tied to your attending's whim. So try to keep your attending happy. Don't suck up. Nothing is worse than that. But do be courteous. And, courtesy starts with promptness. Respect your attending's time even when it might be inconvenient for you or you feel too busy. If you're late and irritate your attending, your whole team will feel the consequence. Hopefully, you'll have a wonderful, understanding attending. There are many of them out there. But even if your attending is understanding, don't antagonize him or her. Show your respect by being on time.

CONSIDER HOW PATIENTS LOOK EVEN WHEN THEY SAY THEY'RE FINE

Don't assume everything is all right solely on the basis of your patients' verbal responses. One of your jobs as an intern will be to hone your clinical skills and intuition. Every patient you see and help manage will mold this intuition. Learning from books, journals, and classroom discussions provides the foundation for your clinical, diagnostic, and management skills. But seeing patients at the bedside on a daily basis will be what turns you into a true clinician. It is sort of like training and drilling to go to war. Once you're in battle, the field conditions are never quite like what you rehearsed. Mike Tyson is not known for his sage rhetoric, but he did have at least one quotable insight. He said, "Everybody's got a plan—until he gets hit."

Remember that books form the backbone of your training, but patients don't always fit nicely into the mold. The exception, rather than the rule, is to see an individual patient who fits precisely the description you've read in books. Rather, each patient represents a nuanced world of his or her own, and you will need to allow yourself a little flexibility in how you approach each of them.

"This patient isn't going to do well tonight." The doctor scratched his chin as he walked out of the room, leading the group of residents and students.

"Why?" asked the senior resident. "Her vitals are stable. We have her on ceftriaxone and azithromycin, which we know are covering her infection, and she feels okay. I think she'll be fine. Probably go home in a couple of days."

The older doctor paused in the hall and looked down at his young students. His eyes glazed over slightly as if lost in thought. Then, he came back and his eyes focused sharply on the resident. "That woman is going to have a bad night. Did you see the way she looked? Go back in there when you have a chance and look at her. Examine her again. She isn't doing as well as you think."

The resident shook his head, dismissing the older doctor's words.

That night the patient spiked a high fever. It took another week and several tests before her doctors learned that she had picked up a fungal infection as well as the bacterial one.

LESSON LEARNED

No amount of book learning can replace clinical experience. Of course, without book learning, clinical experience is simply dangerous. Sometimes, decades of clinical experience can put a physician out of touch with the latest treatments if that physician doesn't keep up with his or her reading. So, being a physician for a longer length of time doesn't mean that physician is necessarily better, but it does mean that he or she has a wealth of experience. It is this experience that you should respect. And, it is this experience that you will begin to accumulate as an intern. As you accumulate experience, learn also to trust your instincts. They will usually lead you in the right direction.

👍 ADMIT IGNORANCE AND THEN DO SOMETHING ABOUT IT

Don't be afraid to say, "I don't know. I'll find out." To many of you, maybe most of you, this is a no-brainer. Still, I have repeatedly seen medical students, interns, and residents alike asked questions that they simply answer with, "I don't know."

✌️ *LESSON LEARNED*

It's not that "I don't know" is an incorrect answer—if you don't know, then you don't know. It's just that adding those three extra words, "I'll find out" makes the answer so much better. "I don't know. I'll find out," shows that you may not know the answer, but you care and are an active learner. If you want to make a good impression then add the "I'll find out." The catch is that then, to really be a rock-star intern, you actually do need to go and find the answer when the pimping is done and report back to your resident or attending with what you find.

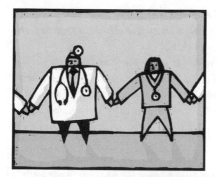

Chapter 4

Staff Relationships: Do's and Don'ts

👍 MAINTAIN A PROFESSIONAL TONE OF VOICE IN THE HOSPITAL

Part of being a doctor means always behaving professionally. Part of behaving professionally is remaining in control. Make it a point to not lose your cool. Yelling is one loud and clear sign that you have most definitely lost your cool. In the world of hospital temperament, yelling at a nurse, patient, or staff member or colleague is like a bright neon blinking sign over your head announcing that you, yes you, are a loose cannon. Don't do it.

The following took place at an urban city hospital.

We were all tired and stressed. It was about a month into internship and we were just getting to know one another.

Angie was one of the interns. The two of us got along well, but I could tell that she had a short fuse. Up until that day, she had kept her temper in check.

A bunch of us were sitting together at lunch. Angie was paged and came back to the table grumbling about being called for trivial things. It was a common complaint from all of us. The nurses on 6 South in particular were notorious for paging about every little thing. A few seconds later Angie got paged again.

I watched her go to the phone and dial. She listened for a couple of seconds and then banged the phone into the wall. "I KNOW SHE HAS A FEVER. THAT'S WHY I ORDERED BLOOD AND URINE CULTURES. THAT'S WHY I ORDERED A CHEST X-RAY. CAN'T YOU READ MY GOD DAMN NOTE?" Angie had lost it. She was screaming into the phone. "WHAT IS WRONG WITH YOU?" She slammed the phone down.

The patients and their families in the cafeteria were all staring at her. She came back to the table and sat down.

One of the interns tried to crack a joke but it fell flat. "Wrong number?"

We were all frustrated with annoying pages, but I never saw anyone lose her cool like Angie did. The rest of us would complain to each other, suffer in silence, talk to the nurses in a reasonable tone, or at least try to deflect our anger with humor. Over the course of the next two months, Angie kept having outbursts. Some of the residents tried talking to her about how to better handle those situations, but it never worked. We started distancing ourselves from her more frequently both literally and figuratively. It became harder to take her seriously as a professional, and no one wanted to be around her when she blew a fuse.

LESSON LEARNED

Not yelling doesn't mean that you can't get angry. It doesn't mean that you shouldn't get angry. It doesn't even mean that you shouldn't express your anger. It just means you shouldn't express your anger or frustration by yelling. Yelling is not an option. If you are upset about something, take a moment to compose yourself and then go to the person who is upsetting you. Whenever possible, take the person aside to a private place and discuss the matter in a direct but controlled manner. If you are concerned about how the interaction might go, you might want to have someone else with you during the confrontation. I want to emphasize that you don't want to be a pushover or be perceived as a pushover. You are, and should be, a leader in the hospital. So act like a good one. Stay calm, assertive, and in control at all times. And, remember, a good leader knows when to lead, when to follow, and when to ask for help. As an intern, you'll be doing a lot of those latter two—but you're still a leader.

DON'T TAKE THINGS PERSONALLY

It's not that business and personal life don't mix at all, but take a lesson from Michael Corleone in *The Godfather* when he said, "It's not personal, Sonny. It's strictly business." Being a hospital employee is stressful and hard work—tempers do flare, nerves run short, and some people just aren't as pleasant or considerate as they could be. Ancillary staff won't treat you with the respect you feel you deserve. Other residents won't be courteous. Attendings will be short with you. It's almost never personal. The following occurred in a large community hospital.

I knew a resident who took everything personally. Any and every small slight became a personal vendetta. In the hospital, that soon added up to a lot of vendettas. He was constantly picking fights. For example, a nurse reprimanded him once for not writing an order quickly enough. He took this personally, and when the nurse forgot something the next day, he yelled at her for negligence. The nurse was so upset that she went to the program director to complain about the resident. As part of her complaint, she catalogued all of the mistakes she knew that the resident had made since starting on the service. The program director called the resident to her office to try and talk some sense into him. He took this personally as well and was convinced that the program director was "against" him.

 LESSON LEARNED

Lighten up. It's hard, but do it anyway. You'll save yourself a lot of hassle. Let small things slide. Everyone is stressed around you in a hospital. Don't get sucked into the personal squabbles. You don't have to be a pushover, but you don't have to go looking for fights, either. Be sensible. If someone seems to be acting inappropriately with you or if someone does something you really think was over the line and a slight, be direct. Tell the person that you don't appreciate being spoken to in such a manner. But, then move on. There are unstable people around you in the workplace just as in life. Be the calm eye of the storm. Your colleagues will like you better, and your life will be much more pleasant and rewarding.

As a quick aside, I remember a patient I had when I was doing a medical school rotation in psychiatry. He was a very successful business man on Wall Street. His earnings were in the high six figures. He polluted himself with cocaine and anger. When he finally realized he had a problem, he started seeing a psychologist. He described driving to see the psychologist and sitting in traffic. He would get so angry about the traffic that he would squeeze the steering wheel until his knuckles were bright white and, occasionally, would pound the seat next to him with his fist. By the time I saw him in the inpatient unit, he had lost much of his money and mellowed some. But I could still envision this large man driving in traffic in a ball of anger just ready to explode.

The point is that this was a very high functioning and successful individual. His colleagues at work, he told me, were completely unaware of his problems. You never know what demons your colleagues and staff are hiding. Let their demons be their own. If they are short-tempered or rude, let that be their problem and not yours. Treat them with good natured respect; you'll find it can be infectious even to some of the most resistant personalities.

CULTIVATE GOOD RELATIONSHIPS WITH NURSES

Don't make enemies with a nurse, ever. I know you've heard this before. I know it's obvious, but some interns and residents, incredibly, still do it. The bottom line is don't piss off the nurses. If you piss off one nurse, by the way, you might as well piss off all of them. Nurses spend a lot of time together, so figure they all know about how you treat any one of them. Be nice to them. You don't have to bring in donuts, though it's not a bad idea to do so. But you do have to be respectful at all times. If you aren't respectful to them simply because you were brought up well, then be respectful out of a sense of self-preservation. The following took place at a medium-sized community hospital.

> *An intern called a nurse "stupid" once for not giving a medication at the correct time. When the nurse explained that she had been busy and was going to give it a few minutes later, the intern told her that she was busy, too, and that the nurse should stop complaining about the workload. When that intern was on call at night, she was woken up constantly. She was reportedly called because a blood glucose was slightly elevated, and the nurse wanted to know if the sliding scale should indeed be used. She was woken up and then told that the page was "a mistake." She was woken up for so many trivial things each time she was on call that she never really got any sleep on call for months. Of course, this intern was in general a disagreeable sort, and so I'm sure she pissed off many nurses for many things. But I think that the "stupid" comment was the straw that broke the camel's back and, consequently, ruined any potentially peaceful night of sleep.*

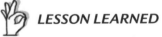 ## LESSON LEARNED

It's really simple. You rely on nurses. They can make your life a lot easier; they can make your life hell; or anything in between. Nurses are the lifeblood of the hospital, your patient's frontline caregivers, and as such they have a lot of power. Furthermore, if you're in a dispute with a nurse, guess whose side your attending physician will likely take? That's right—not yours. Why? Many nurses have held their positions for several years on a particular service and have a prior relationship with your attending. Your attending also knows that they will be there after you are long gone. Remember that your attending didn't survive internship and residency without understanding the importance of our nursing colleagues.

FOSTER CAMARADERIE AND TRUST AMONG YOUR FELLOW INTERNS

The cohesiveness of your intern class will strongly influence and color your internship experience. It can swing either way or anywhere in the middle. Some intern classes forge long-term bonds. After all, it's a bit like boot camp. It's new, hard, rough, exhausting, frustrating, scary, and you all go through it, and grow, together. I did a transitional-year internship, so I went on to a different hospital for my residency training. But I know I will stay close with the intern with whom I did my first general medicine rotation. It wasn't just that we had a good rapport, which we did. But we also looked out for each other. We learned to trust one another. When we ended up working in the ICU together later that year, we covered each other. We lifted each other's spirits when it looked like one of us had had enough.

I remember the movie *The War*, which came out in 1994. Kevin Costner, playing the role of Elijah Wood's father, tells Elijah that if he looked out for his sister, he would always have an ally in the world as they grew up. So it is with internship.

At the other end of the spectrum, some intern classes get downright nasty. The interns don't get along. They are unhappy. Instead of complaining together, they complain about each other. They argue and bicker over small things. Tempers flare. No one looks out for one another, and they even try to get each other in trouble. At one relatively malignant internship, the following story was related to me.

> Simon came up to me and said, "Let's complain about Sathya. The director always has to pick on someone. Let's tell him Sathya's lazy and never does her work."
>
> I couldn't believe what I was hearing. I had never thought of Simon as a bad guy. We had hung out together outside of work, and he had always seemed reasonable. "Are you serious?" I asked him. "Sathya is not a bad worker." In truth, Sathya was annoying, but she worked hard.
>
> Simon could see that I wasn't interested. He shook his head, clearly frustrated, and said, "Never mind. You don't get it." Then I saw him go to someone else and have the same conversation. He didn't have any shame about it at all! He just believed that the director and the senior attendings needed a target, and he wanted to make sure it wasn't going to be him that month.

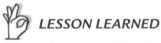 ## LESSON LEARNED

Remember, internship gives you the opportunity to form some organic bonds that you can't manufacture later in life. These bonds can be forged during a few defining times of your life, and this is one of them. Other times might be starting college or going to boot camp. The common thread is a shared purpose and vulnerability at an impressionable time of life, and an important, difficult, and daunting mission ahead.

A more common way that interns squander this opportunity is as follows:

> *"Andy, you look like shit. Rough night?"*
>
> *"Hey Tom, yeah, they kept calling. I sent two patients to the unit. Oh, damn it. I have to present patient Z at morning report and I didn't bring up his x-ray from radiology."*
>
> *"That sucks. Did you eat?" asked Tom.*
>
> *"Are you kidding? I haven't even sat down," replied Andy, shaking his head tiredly and wondering how he was going to get everything done.*
>
> *"Yeah, call sucks. I'm going to go see my patients. See you at morning report."*

✌ LESSON LEARNED

The above happens on an almost daily basis. Can you see anything wrong with it? How could Tom have handled the situation differently? He didn't do anything wrong, per se. It is, after all, how most people act in that situation. But what if Tom had said something like this to Andy: *"Hey, Andy, let me go down and grab that film for you. I'll bring it to report."* Or, how about simply offering: *"I can bring you some breakfast to report. What do you want?"* Can you imagine the good will that Tom would have generated from Andy with these small, easy-to-perform gestures of compassion and kindness? It's really a very small investment on Tom's part but Andy would greatly appreciate it.

When you're post-call, exhausted, defensive from everyone telling you that you forgot something, missed something, or didn't do something right, a kind word or act from a friend or colleague can have a large impact. I still remember the few that were said to me during some of those difficult days, and the faces of those that said them. It is through these small, everyday gestures that strong bonds are formed, or not. Don't squander the opportunity.

As interns, you are going to rely on each other. You will either be strong pillars holding one another up or pushing each other to fall. If you fail to capture this opportunity to stand together, not only will you lose this crucial supporting pillar, but you will also have someone trying to bring you down. More weight bearing down on you is never needed, and it can suffocate you during internship.

This also brings us to don't "dump" on each other. Dumping in internship and residency refers to giving your colleagues work to do that you should have, or could have, rightly done yourself. For example, you have three admissions to do, but you hold one of them until it is after 8 PM so the night float has to do it. Or you sign out to the on-call intern labs that you should have checked during the day. Or you sign out blood draws or any other work. If you dump on your fellow interns, not only will it create bad blood, but they will start dumping on you. By doing your work and helping others do theirs, you will feel better about yourself and, in the long run, it will make your life easier and better. When you are in need of help or a favor, your fellow interns will be that much more likely to lend a helping hand.

AVOID BECOMING A PUSHOVER FOR OTHER INTERNS

You should do what you can to help your fellow interns out. Sometimes, your fellow interns won't seem as apt to help you in return for your goodwill. I encourage you to try anyway. Maybe they just need to warm up to the idea of helping each other out. Maybe they've been burned by coworkers in the past and need to rebuild their trust in relationships. Who knows? But if you go into your relationship with other interns with your fists up, waiting for them to make the first act of good will, you may find yourself waiting a long time. I strongly suggest that you enter with your arms open, expecting the best from them. In my experience, if you give your best and expect their best, you will get it more often than not. The same is true for life in general, but that's another soapbox.

At the same time, remember to set limits. Consider the following example from my own experience.

When I was an intern, a fellow intern named Melanie asked me to cover her floor because she was "very busy." It seemed like an odd request because we were all very busy, but I did it anyway and didn't ask questions. She was nice, and I figured she had her reasons. After all, she knew I was busy, too, so why would she ask me unless it was really important?

A friend of mine in the class came up to me when Melanie walked away and said, "Don't do that, Cooper. Melanie is very clever. She is just taking advantage of you."

I thought about what my friend had said, but I covered Melanie anyway. Still, I filed the warning away in my mind. Melanie never did tell me why she needed my coverage, but that was okay with me. A little while later, Melanie asked me for a similar favor. I obliged, again.

The next week I asked Melanie to help me out with something. She said she really wanted to help but it was a bad time and she was just too overwhelmed. Her husband was upset with her, they had relatives coming in from out of town, and she had to get home as soon as possible. By this time, I had already heard that Melanie had asked someone else to cover her service for an afternoon a month before and was seen by the post-call resident later that day going to a movie with her husband. When Melanie asked me for another favor a few weeks later, I said no.

LESSON LEARNED

Maybe I waited too long to tell Melanie I wasn't interested in always helping her if she was just being lazy. Now, if she really did have a crisis going on, that would have been a different story. But I learned that Melanie just liked to get out of things at the expense of others, and that was not acceptable. The moral here is that you have to find your own limits. Most people in my intern class never helped Melanie. They realized what she was up to and didn't want to spend the energy to find out if Melanie would repay the favor. I think that if you don't try to see the good, you'll always get the bad. But the moral is to set your limits and not be a pushover for your fellow interns. If your intern colleague truly is trying to take advantage of you, don't stand for it.

AVOID BECOMING A PUSHOVER FOR YOUR BOSS

This is a tricky one. First of all, as an intern you will have a lot of "bosses." Your resident is, in some ways, your boss. Your attending is, in some ways, your boss. Your ultimate boss, however, is your residency director. A lot of people will tell you what you should and should not do. Sadly, as an intern you don't have as many rights as you might like. But you do have some rights! Know them and stand up for them when necessary.

Be warned, however, hospitals are political bodies. First and foremost, they are businesses run by administrators. Know when to speak up and when not to. I'll give you an example.

As you probably know or will soon learn, there are federal work-hour regulations for residency programs. Interns and residents are not allowed to work longer than 24 hours at a time. At the time of this writing, resident work hours include the following regulations:

1. *Residents must have at least 10 hours duty-free before returning to work the next day.*
2. *Hours must not exceed 80 hours of work per week, averaged over a 2-week period.*
3. *Residents must not remain on-duty for more than 30 hours, and may not see new patients or cross-cover after 24 hours of duty.*

At one prestigious university hospital, incoming surgical interns are told point-blank that the federal work hour rules are not followed and that they should not expect to work less than 80 hours per week! There is no hiding it there. Interns are told that they are expected to lie about their work hours when the federal regulators come by and ask questions. But, it's all "for the good of the program and in the interest of the residents' education." Amazing.

LESSON LEARNED

In the situation of a program that tells you that they simply don't follow the work hour rules, for example, you have to make a personal decision of whether you want to make a big stink or not. If you do speak up, be forewarned that this is one of those instances in which the nail that sticks up gets hammered down. However, if you can convince your classmates to stand up with you, they will have trouble hammering down all the nails at once. Make your decisions carefully and deliberately, but do know your rights.

> At another internship, the residency program director had a meeting with all of the residents. The interns were violating just about every work-hour rule in the book, and the federal regulators (Joint Commission on the Accreditation of Healthcare Organizations [JCAHO]) were coming to visit. If JCAHO was to find out how the hospital was actually being run, the residency program would likely be put on probation or possibly lose accreditation. The residency director told his residency class the following:
>
> I have a very successful private practice. I'm the chair of this department as well as your director. If you tell the truth and they put the program on probation or close us down, it will affect you much more than me. I don't really care. Think about that when they come to interview you. Tell them you follow the rules.

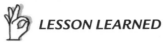 ## LESSON LEARNED

I'm not kidding. This happens all the time. I knew one of the interns in this residency. I was infuriated. My impulse was to call JCAHO myself or maybe even the news press and tell them what was going on. It was, in truth, one of the more malignant internships I had heard of. But, the more I looked into it, the more I learned that the director was correct. If JCAHO came by and the residents told the truth, the ones who would suffer the most if the residency accreditation was revoked would be the residents themselves! It seemed cruel and unfair. It was both of those things, as well as the reality. I think that abuses of work hours are a travesty at many levels, not the least of which is the way they put patients at serious risk, as well as putting interns at risk. I encourage you to always tell the truth to JCAHO, but do be aware of this problem in the system.

On another level, even in a program with a caring director, you may sometimes feel that you are being treated unfairly compared with other interns in your department. Maybe you have more calls or an extra ICU rotation. Don't be a pushover. In a respectful but direct manner, don't be afraid to stand up for yourself. Tell the chief resident if you think the schedule is not fair. Don't expect to be treated better than your classmates, but do expect equity within the program.

AVOID BECOMING A PUSHOVER FOR NURSES

Okay, this is a touchy one. As I mentioned, you should never, ever piss off nurses. But, you shouldn't be a pushover for them, either. Treat them with respect and professionalism, and almost all of them will return the favor. Still, you must watch out for the few that don't. When I was a resident, I had the following conversation with an intern I was close to at another hospital.

> *"Grant, they keep on calling me to come and draw the bloods. There is this one nurse on Madison South who can't find veins on any of her patients. She calls me all the time."*

95

"What happens when she calls you?" I asked. "What do you say?"

"I ask her what's wrong, and she says that she tried three times to get the blood but couldn't. Then she asks me to come and do it."

"What then?"

"I go and draw the blood. Sometimes they're hard sticks, but usually they're easy. The real trouble is that it takes time, and I have other patients I'm covering who are really sick and need my attention."

It was clear that my friend was being taken advantage of. I had heard of this happening before at other places. I told my friend to tell the nurse, the next time she called, that he was busy and she should call her nursing supervisor. If the nursing supervisor couldn't draw the blood or find someone who could, then he would draw it when he finished what he was doing.

My friend implemented the above strategy. The nurse called two more times and each time my friend told her to call the nursing supervisor for help. After the second call, he never got another call from that nurse for help with a blood draw.

LESSON LEARNED

On a more egregious, and probably an illegal, discriminatory, level, I have heard of interns being called to draw disproportionately more bloods from HIV patients than non-HIV patients. From these reports, it is not that the HIV patients are more difficult sticks. This is unacceptable behavior. Depending on your hospital policy, you should be ready to help out with blood draws and other minor procedures. But watch out for being taken advantage of. Most nurses are extraordinary, gifted people who want to help you as well as their patients. If you treat them well, they will do the same for you. But, as in any profession, there are a few bad apples. So be warned and don't be a pushover.

TRY TO LEARN AND USE AS MANY PEOPLE'S NAMES IN THE HOSPITAL AS POSSIBLE, INCLUDING THOSE OF YOUR PATIENTS

This is a bit of colloquial wisdom, I know, and it applies not just to the hospital but to all facets of life. Learn people's names. Some people are naturally better at this than others. Once my wife learns a name, for example, she always remembers it. Watching her, it seems effortless. For me, however, remembering people's names is a skill that I have to work at. I remember faces, and I remember things about people, but somehow names don't stick in my mind. So I make it a point to work on this skill, and I've gotten much better at it.

People like hearing their names. After all, it's *theirs*. Using someone's name is a personal experience. It's an intimate gesture between two people. In a large hospital, probably as in any large business where so much becomes impersonal and people feel slighted and often dehumanized and devalued, using a person's name with the correct pronunciation is appreciated all the more.

It doesn't take much to use a person's name. Instead of, "Hey," or "Um, excuse me, could you . . .", you say, "Excuse me, Doris," etc. I encourage you to learn and use the names of your coworkers in the hospital. For one, it will make your coworkers feel more appreciated.

97

If that's not enough (though hopefully it would be), they will also be more responsive to helping you. The person will understand that you value him or her as a person and not just as an attending physician, a janitor, a clerk, a resident, a medical student, a nurse, or a security guard. You are showing that you care enough about that person to learn and remember his or her name. It is a sign of respect, and people respond to it. I know I do.

So how do you learn and cultivate this skill? Start by introducing yourself. When the other person volunteers his or her name, use it soon and often during your conversation. If you think you might forget the name later, say up front that you are horrible with names and may ask for their name again. When you walk away, repeat their name once or twice in your head and try to consciously associate their name with something distinctive about them.

Using names is important when addressing your patients as well. If a name is difficult to pronounce, ask the patient if you are pronouncing it correctly. Then, use the patient's name as often as you can during the conversation with him or her. Patients will appreciate that you care, and that you think of them as individuals, not just some guy with stomach pain or a bad leg.

An attending once told me that he spent a whole initial interview with a person, taking a full history and physical, and then later discovered that he had been calling the patient by the wrong *name during the whole encounter. The doctor had just made a mistake and gotten the name mixed up. The patient was so intimidated by being in a doctor's office that he hadn't wanted to correct him.*

LESSON LEARNED

Keep this in mind when you are talking with patients. There is a power imbalance. There shouldn't be, but there is. Be aware of this potential inequity and make sure you go out of your way to show the proper respect for your patients. That begins with using their names and pronouncing them correctly.

REPORT SEXUAL, RACIAL, OR ANY OTHER KIND OF DISCRIMINATION

I grew up in Princeton, New Jersey, a small college town. If there was discrimination in Princeton, I never saw it. There were people from all walks of life, of all colors, religions, shapes, and sizes, and we all seemed to get along just fine. I never saw someone put down because of his or her religion or race. I thought that discrimination was the stuff of movies, things that happened in the distant past, or something that happened only in a few backward places left in the world. Of course, I was wrong.

When I was in 5th grade, I went off to a soccer camp in central Jersey. My mother, being a mom, worried about me. I asked my dad why my mom was worried. My dad said that Mom was concerned that other people might give me a hard time because I was Jewish. I laughed. That was the strangest thing I had ever heard. I had grown up with stories of my parents and grandparents facing all sorts of discrimination, but that was in the past, right?

I had a great time at soccer camp. It wasn't until the last two days that things turned ugly. One of the bigger kids got

99

angry about something and used an utterly reprehensible racial slur on one of the smaller African-American kids. I had never heard anyone speak that way. I immediately told the coach, who chuckled and told the older kid to stop. But it was clear that the coach wasn't going to make him. Then some of the other kids joined in. Other races and ethnicities were slurred. It was an incredibly ugly scene. It opened my eyes to a world I wished didn't exist but realized was more real than I had thought.

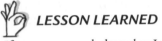 ## LESSON LEARNED

If you grew up sheltered as I did, or if you have been for-tunate to not experience any discrimination, you are lucky, and I hope your luck will continue. Unfortu-nately, discrimination lurks in the hospital just as much as anywhere else. I know of people who have faced sexual discrimination, sexual assault, racial and religious discrimination in the hospital. It is rare, to be sure, but it is there. Be aware of it and don't tolerate an ounce of it. If you see someone else being discriminated against, don't tolerate that, either. Edmund Burke, the 18th-century Anglo-Irish statesman, once said, "All that is necessary for the triumph of evil is that good men do nothing." That statement couldn't be more true, and it goes for you women, too. If you see discrim-ination, speak up. If it happens to you, speak up. Don't wait. There are mechanisms in place in your hospital for complaints and to protect you while making them. Whether the discrimination is coming from the chair-man, program director, janitor, attending, nurse, resident, fellow intern, patient, or president of your hospital, speak up, and make yourself heard.

👍 HELP MAINTAIN AN INOFFENSIVE WORKPLACE ENVIRONMENT

Don't tell dirty jokes to people who might not want to hear them. This seems obvious, but interns, like so many others, sometimes do it nonetheless. There are many stories of interns telling dirty jokes to the wrong people and then getting reprimanded. Whether or not you think dirty jokes are funny, you should at least have enough common sense to know that some people find them offensive. It's not fair to burden them with your vulgarity, so don't do it. If you're going to tell dirty jokes or make off-color remarks, you had better be absolutely sure that your audience wants to hear them. Not only that, but make sure you don't have any unintended audience hanging around. Think before you speak.

To be fair, telling dirty jokes to people who don't want to hear them is not a mistake unique to interns. Not by any means. Lawsuits have likely been filed in all manners of professions for this lapse of judgment. But as an intern, you may be entering the workforce for the first time and so it's important for you to understand that the rules are changing. Things that might have been tolerated in school are no longer tolerated. Be aware of the people around you and be sensitive to their tastes. If you don't, your coworkers might not only find you insensitive, but they may also file a complaint or a lawsuit against you.

👍 SHOW RESPECT TO EVERYONE IN THE HOSPITAL

Showing respect reflects how you were raised. I often recall a lesson from my father.

101

I was in middle school, and my father was on the local school board. I went with my mother to pick him up after one of the board meetings. At the end of the meeting, there were a lot of people milling around discussing things. I was standing with my father. Leroy, one of the custodial workers, came up to my father and said, "I had them make the chocolate chip ones you like." I looked down and saw a large plate of freshly baked chocolate chip cookies. My father smiled. "Thanks, Leroy. This is my son." We shook hands.

When Leroy walked away, I asked my father if he and Leroy were friends. "No," my father said, "Not really. But I've known him for a long time. He's a good man. Treat people as you want to be treated, Grant. You will always get what you give."

The best sermons are seen, not heard.

LESSON LEARNED

A hospital is a large, living, breathing entity. There are many people involved in its intricate workings. If you don't treat people with respect because it's the right thing, then at least do it because it will make your life easier with the nursing staff, help you get the forms you need from the administrative staff, help you get fresh white coats when yours get too dirty, help you get food from the cafeteria when you forgot your wallet and your meal card has run out, and innumerable other small things that make your day easier and more pleasant. When you're an intern, you need help from a lot of people. Treating people with respect is a must if you hope to receive it in return.

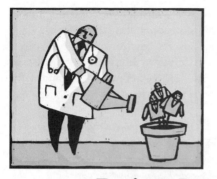

Chapter 5

Patient Interactions: Do's and Don'ts

👍 BE COMPASSIONATE WHEN TELLING SOMEONE THAT A LOVED ONE HAS DIED

Death is a part of life, and it is something that you will have to get used to as an intern. Everyone handles this differently. What I think is most important is to realize that some of your patients will die, and there is nothing you can do about it. It was just their time. You do what you can to make them better, but sometimes you can't do enough. That's not your fault. It's the cycle of life.

As part of coming to terms with death in the hospital, you will also have to help others come to terms with it. One of your jobs will be to inform family members that their grandparent, parent, sibling, child, or significant

103

other has passed on. You will likely have to do this so many times that it will become almost routine. I urge you, however, to remember that no matter how often you have done so, it is definitely not routine to the person receiving the news. Don't become nonchalant. In this story, I offer my own experience.

The first time I had to tell a family member that a loved one had died, it was 3 AM. The nurse from the oncology floor woke me and asked me to pronounce a patient dead. I had only been an intern for a few weeks, and no one had prepared me for this inevitability. My friend was sleeping in the bunk bed next to mine and the call had woken him as well. (Later we'll talk about why you don't share a call room if possible!) My friend shrugged when I asked him how you pronounce someone dead. He hadn't pronounced anyone yet, either. He sleepily told me to look in one of the books he kept in his pocket for the page on pronouncing. I did so and proceeded to the oncology floor.

When I arrived at the patient's bedside, it was clear that the spark of life was no longer within him. At the time, I was sure I would never forget the face of the first man I pronounced dead. I remember he was a thin, elderly Caucasian with sparse gray hair. But, to be honest, through the fog of the numerous other intense experiences I had in internship and residency, I can no longer picture him more than that.

While it was clear that he was dead, I wanted to do things right. After all, what if he wasn't dead after all? I had to be sure, and I wanted to do it by the book. I did a sternal rub. I pinched his fingers, checked his pulse, flashed a light in his pupils, and listened for heart sounds and breath sounds. He was dead. I felt bad rubbing his sternum. It seemed somehow wrong to disturb this lifeless man by trying to hurt him. I pronounced him and made a note of the time. In the stillness of the late hour, I stood in the room and wondered what this was all about. Is this how life was supposed to end—in a cold hospital room, alone, with only a stranger's face in a white coat poking and prodding you to make sure you wouldn't somehow wake up and come alive again?

I went to the nurse's station and wrote a note in his chart. Then I asked the nurse if there was anything else I was supposed to do. "Call the family," was her reply. Call the family. I wasn't even this man's doctor. I didn't know his family. Shouldn't his oncologist be calling? But, at 3:30 AM, the job fell to me. I found the number I was supposed to call and then, after trying to figure out how to tell the person at the other end of the line what I had to tell him or her, I dialed.

A woman's voice answered the phone. I placed her at about 40 years old. I told her my name and where I was calling from. I asked her how she knew the patient. He was her father. "I have some bad news to tell you." Then I told her that her father had died. There was a pause and then the voice at the other end of the line said:

"Oh, okay, thanks for calling. We were expecting this."

She didn't sound frantic. She sounded like a loving daughter who had come to peace with what she knew was close at hand. I was, frankly, relieved. I hadn't known what to expect. Would she scream, cry, yell, deny? I had no idea

About a week later, I received a similar call around 4 AM. Another patient on the oncology floor had died. This time, I was prepared. For one, I had experienced it already. For another, I had talked with other residents in the interim and found out that, on average, we would be called to pronounce a patient on the oncology floor about once a week because many of the patients were on comfort care.

I went to the patient's room. I wouldn't say I was at ease with the idea of going through the pronouncing again, but at

105

least I felt more confident with what I had to do and what to expect. The patient's wife answered the phone. I told her, as I had told the other patient's daughter the previous week, who I was and that I had bad news. When I told her that her husband had died quietly and peacefully in his room, she shrieked. Then she cried. My heart dropped. "I thought we had more time," she told me. "What happened?" I was not prepared for this. I told her how sorry I was for her loss.

Immediately, when I heard the wife's reaction, I started wondering if I could have phrased my news to her differently. I wondered if I had rushed telling her. Might I have done things differently? In the moment, and ever since, I have thought so.

LESSON LEARNED

It's really hard to learn how to tell someone that a loved one has died, and even harder to do it well. I don't profess by any means to have the answers how. There probably is no best way. In the end, you still have the same awful news. But there are ways to finesse it—to give family members a few extra moments to brace themselves, particularly when it's unexpected news. They will probably have a hard time processing all that you tell them. Unfortunately, practice is really needed to get better. But, the moral of this story is don't be nonchalant about it. What I learned was to brace myself each time before telling the loved one. Remind yourself what a profoundly important moment this is for him or her. If you remind yourself of that, and you do your utmost to take your time and be empathetic, you will at least have done your best, and that is all anyone, including you, can ask of you. So, learn from my mistake. No matter how many times you do it, remember to take your time and respect the moment. Sometimes you'll pronounce patients who seem like they have been at death's doorstep for months or years. You'll expect the family members to have anticipated the death. They might have. But they might not have. Don't assume. Tell them the way you would want to be told. Be direct, but always compassionate.

GIVE YOUR PATIENTS THE BENEFIT OF THE DOUBT

Don't assume that just because your patient isn't following your instructions that he or she is difficult or even demented. This happens more often than you'd like to think. The following story illustrates the potential of this mistake.

> *An elderly Chinese man was admitted to the hospital with fever, chills, and lethargy. At first, his doctors were unable to get a medical history because they believed the man only spoke Chinese. When a translator was brought in, the man still couldn't communicate so it was believed that he had perhaps suffered a brain injury and was aphasic. About two weeks into his hospital admission, someone was struck with the insight that maybe the man was hard of hearing! So he was, and after a hearing aid was obtained, his doctors were finally able to interview him.*

LESSON LEARNED

The moral here is obvious: Never assume. Many patients are only slightly hard of hearing, so they may hear enough to understand some of what you say but miss other words. Particularly in a hospital setting, where patients have enough trouble understanding what you're saying when their hearing is intact, this can be a problem. If you have any doubt about your patient's ability to hear and/or understand you, there is a simple, inexpensive test to find out. Ask them! It's an amazingly effective approach.

 ## USE STRAIGHTFORWARD, CLEAR LANGUAGE WHEN TALKING ABOUT DEATH AND CANCER

Avoid euphemisms about death. Don't tell someone that a loved one has "passed on" or "gone to a better place." If a patient has died, you need to tell the loved one that the patient has "died" or is "dead." You have to use the word. A resident related to me the following incident that took place when he was an intern.

> *I came out of the code and told the guy's wife that I had bad news. I told her that we had done everything we could to save him, but in the end we couldn't. He was at peace now. The wife nodded and said she understood. I asked her if she had other family members or anyone she wanted me to call. "My daughter is waiting for me to call."*
>
> *"Would you like a phone?"*
>
> *"Oh, no, not right now."*
>
> *"I understand." I thought she wanted some time to pre-pare herself. I was about to ask her if she wanted to see her husband's body when she said,*
>
> *"When will John be waking up? I'd like to see him to see how he is doing so I can tell my daughter when I talk to her."*

LESSON LEARNED

Sometimes, it is not clear why misunderstandings happen. In the above scenario, it *seems* clear that the intern was telling the patient's wife her husband had died. But, unless you use the word, you run the risk of being misunderstood, which is unacceptable. The same goes for telling someone that he or she has cancer. If you have to relay that information, at some point in the conversation you have to use the word "cancer." If you spend the whole conversation talking about a malignancy or a tumor, you run the risk of a misunderstanding. It happens all the time. Realize that some words will hit home. Use them gently, but use them. Someone might misunderstand "passed on," "gone to a better place," or "is at peace." But no one misunderstands "dead." For the same reason you feel uncomfortable saying it, you need to say it.

USE THERAPEUTIC TOUCH ON YOUR PATIENTS WHEN APPROPRIATE

Don't underestimate the value of holding your patient's hand. The power of touch and the ability of touch to heal can be profound. Consider what you already know—that infants grow more when they are loved and held. I want to use this section to encourage you to not fear your patients, and to touch them.

When she was in high school, my wife used to volunteer at the local hospital. That is probably why I also volunteered at the local hospital, but that's another story. One day, she was

109

helping out in the emergency room. A nurse saw her candy-striped uniform and earnest, pretty face. She approached Ana and asked if she would mind sitting with an old woman in cubicle three. She was dying, the nurse explained, and had no family with her. Ana obliged and sat down next to her. She didn't know quite what to say to her, or even if the dying woman could see or hear her. But she held her hand until it was time for her to go home. The next day, the dying woman was gone. Ana can still remember the way the old woman's frail, withered hand felt in her own young, pink, healthy one. She hoped the old woman had found some comfort in not dying alone.

LESSON LEARNED

Some people are naturally more "touchy-feely" than others. Whether you are or not, though, try holding your patient's hand. Let patients know you aren't afraid of them. Even when it's late, even when the room has the scent of urine wafting in the air—maybe especially when this is the case—and you can't remember all of their lab values, and you don't know why a certain test is being done but you have to ask them a question— pause and look them in the eyes and hold their hands while you talk to them. Feel their humanity, and let it evoke your own.

In the hospital, remember that your patient is probably scared. There is a power differential between you and the patient. There shouldn't be, but there is. Your patient is sick, and you are not. Your patient doesn't understand what is going on to his or her body, and you do. Your patient takes the medications that you prescribe. Part of your job is to empower your patient as much as you can by educating him or her. But, acknowledge that a certain amount of fear may still exist, and acknowledge that you have the ability to alleviate some of that fear by simply reaching out, literally as well as figuratively.

Your patient listens to what you say, but also reads your body language. Even if you say the most comforting words, if your body language says something different, your patient will most likely respond to your body language. If you lean away from your patient, he or she will notice. Likewise, if you show you are unafraid, if you show that you care, if you hold his or her hand, your patient will notice that, too.

Consider, also, that you will likely one day have your own outpatient office. Your success in this office will have as much to do with your ability to relate to people as it will with your clinical acumen. Learning to relate to people, if it doesn't come naturally to you, is part of your training. Holding hands is a good place to start.

USE A TRANSLATOR IF YOU DON'T SPEAK THE SAME LANGUAGE AS YOUR PATIENT

If your patient only speaks a foreign language, don't just talk more loudly in English and expect him or her to understand you. I wouldn't have included this one, because it seems so obvious, but a colleague told me this story from her internship, and two others confirmed similar but distinct experiences in their respective residencies, so into the book it goes.

111

We were rounding with two other teams and we came across a pleasant-looking patient from Japan. There was a sea of white coats, and we all crowded into the patient's small room. It was one of those terrible rounds when there are so many of you that some of you end up huddled around the patient's roommate's bed because there is not enough room for everyone. In fact, a couple of people spilled out into the hallway for want of space. Anyway, there we were. The intern who was presenting was named Kate.

Kate was a tall woman. She was a little older than most of the other interns and had a voice that projected well. Because she was so tall, I could see her even though I was toward the back of the group.

"This is Ms. C.," I heard Kate say. "She is a 73-year-old . . ." Kate proceeded to give a brief, well-organized description of Ms. C. When she was finished, the attending nodded and said, "Okay, Kate, good job. Ms. C, how are you doing?" The attending asked the patient.

"Oh," Kate jumped in. "Her English is not very good. Her husband usually translates." "Ms. C," Kate turned to the patient, raising her voice, "HOW ARE YOU DOING?"

I couldn't see the patient from behind the crowd, but she didn't say anything. Then, the attending tried again. "MS. C, HOW . . . ARE . . . YOU . . . DOING?" She spoke loudly and slowly and enunciated clearly.

I moved my head and spotted the patient through the army of white coats in front of me. She shook her head apologetically and with a sheepish grin, said, "No English," just loud enough for me to hear in the back of the room.

A snicker broke out from one of the residents in front of me. The attending either heard the snicker or realized the futility and absurdity of speaking more loudly and slowly. The attending asked, "Could one of you get a translator on the phone?"

112

✋ *LESSON LEARNED*

We should all know that talking more loudly and slowly to a patient who does not speak our language is not going to increase the patient's understanding of it. Know whether your patient understands and speaks English. If not, and if you don't speak your patient's language, then get a translator. It is obvious, and I make the point not to be condescending, but because sometimes, perhaps through the seemingly endless hours, common sense gets checked at the door. And, as you can see from this example, not just interns, but attendings face this problem as well.

👍 KEEP THE LEVEL OF YOUR INTERACTION WITH YOUR PATIENTS PROFESSIONAL

Don't "hit on" your patients. By the time you get to internship, you have probably been warned that it is inappropriate and unacceptable to have a romantic relationship with your patients. If you haven't, let me be the first to tell you. If you have, let me reinforce it, "loud and clear." Don't "come on" to your patients. There are no exceptions to this rule. Despite this, I have heard many reports of inappropriate behavior. The following story was reported by one intern who overheard another.

I went over her x-ray with her and told her that because she was only having her arm set, and wasn't really sick, it would be okay for us to go out together. She gave me her digits.

113

✌️ *LESSON LEARNED*

This is not acceptable. If you see your colleagues hitting on their patients, report them. As a physician, you are in a position of power over your patients and to hit on them is to exploit them. That goes for women as well as men. Popular television shows about doctors depict young interns and residents falling in love with their patients all the time (e.g., *Scrubs, Grey's Anatomy*). That's television, not reality. Don't do it. No exceptions.

👍 SPEAK RESPECTFULLY TO YOUR PATIENTS

How do you speak with your patients? How do you balance being respectful, using very simple language, and not being condescending? Your patient may be sick, but that doesn't make him or her mentally impaired. At the same time, your patients are likely to be at least somewhat overwhelmed by the hospital experience and trying to understand exactly what is happening to their bodies, and what you and the other doctors are doing to make them better. Being sick in the hospital is a lot to take in.

If you talk to your patients as if they are children, you are patronizing them. Then again, if you use big words or, worse, medical jargon, you risk them not understanding you, which will add to their anxiety. These are things that no one ever really teaches you. Sure, some physicians might have mentioned it to you. But, mostly you learn by imitating the physicians around you, who likely followed the examples of the physicians around them. Sometimes, you get stuck in a situation in which you don't find good role models and you see what *not* to do. This makes things more difficult. A few general guidelines can always be used for how to talk with your patients.

First of all, make good eye contact. If you can't make good eye contact, your patient will assume that you are either hiding something or you lack confidence. Do look your patient directly in the eye. Good communication starts with good eye contact.

Do speak slowly and distinctly. You are not at home. Don't mumble. A slow cadence of speech transmits calmness and confidence.

Even if your patient has a PhD in biochemistry, don't use medical jargon. If you can't explain something using everyday language that a 6th grader could understand, then you don't really understand it. You might get away with using medical jargon to explain something. Your patient might look at you, nod, and say that he or she understands, but that doesn't necessarily mean that he or she really does, and it doesn't mean that you do either. This doesn't take much effort. Sometimes, it's as easy as saying, "Your heart is not pumping well, and so the fluid is getting backed up into your lungs and making it hard to breathe. We're going to give you a water pill so that you pee out some of the extra fluid. And we're also going to give you two medications to make it easier for your heart to pump the fluid through your body." This is much more helpful than saying, "You have left ventricular failure, which is why you are having so much dyspnea. We're going to give you a diuretic, an ACE inhibitor, and a beta blocker." Your patient will appreciate your being able to express yourself in language that is easy for them to relate to. As you talk to them, you may alter the level of your communication. Often, I think it is useful and respectful to explain briefly in medical terminology, followed quickly by saying something like, "In English, what that means is . . ."

Just remember that when it comes to talking about someone's body, emotion will cloud his or her understanding of what you are saying. In a normal, everyday conversation, it may be acceptable to not understand or hear every part of what is being said, but in a hospital, between patient and physician, you should aim for full comprehension. Even if your patient is a physician, still keep the medical jargon to a minimum. A 68-year-old psychiatrist may not be up on the latest oncology jargon.

Likewise, don't, under any circumstances, make baby sounds when talking to or encouraging an adult patient. I've never seen a nurse do this, but I have seen and heard doctors and therapists do it. I don't understand it. Would you want someone cooing over you? Encourage adults with adult language and adult sounds. Leave baby voices and prolonged "ooohhhs" and "aaahhhhhs" for the nursery and pediatric patients.

I once did a consult on a patient who had been labeled a rich, spoiled person who wanted everything "her way." When I met with her, we instantly hit it off. She wasn't difficult, she just didn't like it when the therapists "oooohhhed" and "aaahhh-hed" when she got up and took a few steps. The therapists complained that the patient wasn't being cooperative, and the physicians labeled her noncompliant. She was neither. She just wanted to be treated with dignity and respect.

116

LESSON LEARNED

Speak to others as you would want to be spoken to. If you were 74 years old and in the hospital with a cardiac condition, how would you respond to a 27-year-old doctor using baby talk? Even if it's well-intentioned, using baby talk demeans adult patients and it makes you look . . . well . . . it makes you look like a grown-up talking baby talk to an elder. Preserve your own dignity by helping them preserve theirs. Treat them with respect, and speak to them as an adult.

APPRECIATE THE SANCTITY OF INDIVIDUAL LIFE

Even when you're swamped with patients; even when you know death is inevitable for a patient; don't rejoice over your patient's death—ever. Internship and residency are taxing and demanding. Sometimes, you are taking care of so many patients that you have trouble keeping up. When this happens, you just want your patients off your service. However, no matter how much you may want them to go away; no matter how much you may yearn for them to just leave, never yearn for them to die. Consider the following story, which took place in a small, community hospital. Steve is an intern on the same service as the intern telling the story.

I couldn't believe what Steve said one time. We were rounding one morning with our senior resident and came to Steve's patient Mr. Y. We couldn't find him and finally we went to the clerk.

"Oh, Mr. Y," the clerk told us, "he died last night. They just took his body out."

"Yeeessss!" Steve exclaimed as he pumped his fist in the air. "One less patient."

I looked at Paula, our senior resident. She was looking in disbelief at Steve who was excitedly crossing off Mr. Y's name from his list.

For some time, I couldn't get that image out of my head. Steve, ecstatic that his patient had died, pumping his fist in the air.

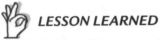 ## LESSON LEARNED

In all likelihood, Steve wasn't a "bad guy." He had probably come to think of his patients not as humans, but rather as diagnoses. The pancreatic cancer that keeps asking for more pain meds. Not Mr. Y, husband and father of six, lover of dogs and boats. No, he was pancreatic cancer in room 334A.

Don't be like Steve. Remember whom you are treating. Remember that they have names and families. I hope that Paula sat down with Steve and put him straight. His behavior was simply and obviously unacceptable. No matter how tired you get, no matter how overworked you feel, remember your humanity and that of your patients.

RESPECT YOUR PATIENTS' TIME AND PRIVACY

Show respect for your patients and do so with grace. Answers.com defines "grace" as "seemingly effortless beauty or charm of movement, form, or proportion. A characteristic or quality pleasing for its charm or refinement. A sense of fitness or propriety."

One of my professors in medical school said to us once, during our first year, that we were all going to get through school and become doctors, but that we should try to do it with a little bit of grace. *Do it with grace.* He was not my favorite professor, but I always remembered that advice as some of the best ever given.

Part of grace is the way we treat other people. To that end, another attending physician gave some helpful advice.

"Always thank people for their time," he told me. And he did. Whenever he went to see a patient in the hospital, at the end of it he would thank that patient for his or her time. Patients in the hospital are always at someone else's mercy for their daily schedule. They have to wait for breakfast, wait for lunch, wait for their x-ray—even wait for someone to take them to the bathroom. No one ever thinks about their time. "How would that make you feel?" he would ask me.

LESSON LEARNED

Thanking patients for their time is a simple, humane courtesy. They are giving us access to their bodies, their internal organs and flesh, their fears and their souls, all with the hope that we can help them. The least we can do is say thank you. I don't always do it, by the way. It depends on the situation. Sometimes I do, but at other times it seems overly solicitous. Regardless, I think it's a good attitude to keep in your mind and outlook. This is their time, too.

Privacy is another thing that patients lose to a varying extent in the hospital and the outpatient office. Of course, some parts of privacy require sacrificing. Lungs must be listened to; rectals must at times be performed. But, that doesn't mean that we can't at least try to preserve as much privacy as possible. If you are not examining a part of the body, keep it covered. If you need to get an extra sheet, do that. Sometimes, the attempt is as valuable as the result.

> *An attending who was practicing sports medicine would always have the patient in a gown when doing a back exam. One particularly large patient didn't quite fit within the gown. While doing a reverse straight leg raise with the patient lying on her stomach, the gown did little to offer privacy. He took a sheet from the stack and covered her. The sheet kept slipping. The patient said, "That's all right. I don't mind." The attending responded, "No, no. We don't always get it right, but we can at least try to keep your privacy." As he put the sheet back on her, I saw her face, and I could tell that what she appreciated even more than the attending keeping her covered was that he valued her as a person and respected her dignity.*

LESSON LEARNED

Webster's online dictionary defines grace as "The exercise of love, kindness, mercy, favor; disposition to benefit or serve another; favor bestowed or privilege conferred." Another definition as it applies to the hospital, at least a working definition, might be, "The showing of dignity and respect, with love and kindness in your heart and humility for your task." I think we'd be better off if we could all remember that.

DON'T DRINK OR EAT WHILE TREATING PATIENTS

As far as 99% of your attendings are concerned, this is a major no-no. It smacks of unprofessionalism. Don't do it.

I'd like to add the counter argument, though, that under certain circumstances, it may possibly be acceptable. Those circumstances are in the outpatient setting and only if you can offer your patient something to eat or drink as well. My wife spent some time in Holland working with a famous dance medicine physician. This physician had a wonderful practice, and he would offer tea to his patients. I don't think it gets much more civilized. Still, for most of the time, and for 100% of the time while you're an intern in the hospital, don't eat or drink (and that includes coffee) while talking or meeting with your patients.

ANSWER PATIENT QUESTIONS ACCURATELY AND HONESTLY

If a patient asks you a question and you are unsure of the answer, don't just guess. Maybe this one is obvious, and maybe it's not. Even when you are a medical student, patients often expect you to know as much about their care as the attending physician does. When they look at you, they may not see a student, they just see a white coat and probably don't realize the significance of its length. As an intern, you will be introducing yourself as a doctor, and so this effect becomes magnified. Patients will assume that you are informed about their pathologies, their medical care, and their prognosis. If they ask you a question and you answer it, they won't think that you're guessing. They won't be able to distinguish you as the junior person on the team who might not know what's going on with all their problems. To the contrary, they will expect that your statements are correct. If you give them your guess, they will have every reason to think it's also their primary care doctor's guess. So, be careful about what you say. The following is a benign example that was related to me and took place in a large, prestigious university hospital.

> *I was making my rounds when Ms. G asked me if she was going to need a valve replacement. I told her that, from my understanding, she would probably need one sooner than later, almost definitely within the year. She seemed to accept this. Later, when I rounded with my attending, he told her that she would not need a valve for several years. Ms. G looked extremely confused and protested that I had told her she would need one within the year. She didn't want one, she assured us, but didn't know whom to believe. It took another 20 minutes of my attending's time to undo the confusion I had caused.*

 LESSON LEARNED

You can and should talk to your patients about what you do know about their care. I also think that you can tell them what you *think but aren't sure of.* But, to be fair to the patient, I believe you have to be very careful to explain how junior you are and that the attending may have very different ideas about what is going on. In the end, it is good practice for you to get in the habit of talking to your patients about their diseases, but it's also only fair to explain to your patients how many cases you have seen and your level of training. Finally, always realize that many patients, no matter how much explaining you do, won't really understand that you may not know what is going on in your attending's head when it comes to an individual patient's care.

AVOID TELLING YOUR PATIENT "SEE YOU LATER," IF YOU KNOW YOU PROBABLY WON'T

We've all probably been guilty of this at some time or another. It's often easier to say, "See you later," than it is to say "Goodbye." Have you ever noticed that some people even say "See you later," to those people they know they have very little chance of *ever* seeing again? For example, they'll say it to the *maître d'* as they leave a restaurant in a state they are only passing through.

Saying "See you later" without really meaning it is so common, in fact, that the online Urban Dictionary defines the term as being equivalent to: "good bye . . . (it) does not imply that another encounter will actually ever happen." In the hospital, however, it's another story. The following story is my own.

> I used to say "See you later," without thinking about it. It was part of my vernacular that I picked up in either high school or college. I never really thought about it until my internship. While in the elevator, an older woman smiled at me so I smiled back. I didn't recognize her at all.
>
> "You don't recognize me, do you?"
>
> "No," I confessed. "Have we met?"
>
> "You saw me in the hospital with a group of doctors. You told me you would see me later but then I never saw you again."
>
> I studied her face. Who was she? I couldn't place her. "I'm sorry," I said, "I don't remember. Which floor were you on?"
>
> "I was on the fifth floor."
>
> I remembered. Not her name, but I remembered when I had seen her. She was a patient on a team I was covering for the day. I didn't remember telling her that I would see her later, but that didn't mean a thing. Often, when I would leave

123

*a room, I would smile and tell the patient I would see him or
her later. Usually, I did, but it never crossed my mind that if I
didn't see the patient again that it would be a problem or
cause any confusion. I had seen this woman once, and she had
remembered that I had said, "See you later."*

LESSON LEARNED

If you've ever been a patient in the hospital, you know it
can be an intimidating experience. You don't have control over things. You eat when the food comes. You go
to the bathroom when the nurse brings a commode.
You depend on your doctors and nurses to take care of
you. If you're not a doctor or familiar with the way hospitals work, you don't know which doctor is in charge,
which one is the intern just trying to figure out the
computer system, and which one is a consultant. Some
medical students are introduced as "doctor." It's confusing for patients.

When a doctor says "See you later," patients may
actually expect to see them later. When the doctor
doesn't return, the patients may feel abandoned or
think that the doctor forgot about them. It's not fair
to patients to risk this miscommunication. Start
training yourself now to say things like "Goodbye," or,
"It was nice to meet you. Have a good night," instead
of "See you later." It took me a while, but if I can do it,
then so can you.

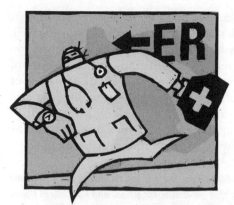

Chapter 6

On Call: Do's and Don'ts

👍 **ATTEND TO YOUR PAGER**

If you're like me, at some point in your life you might have thought it would be cool to have a pager. Maybe you were in a restaurant and saw someone, presumably a doctor, get up to answer a page and you wondered what important business that person had to attend to. In any case, if you are like me, and like most interns, you might find yourself at some point during internship wondering what would happen if you just chucked your pager off the roof. Or, more mildly, what would happen if you just didn't answer your pager?

Would the world come to an end if you didn't answer your pager? Would the walls implode? Would a

125

life end? Would someone lie needlessly in pain? Or would the work somehow get done without you? Well, if you are indeed like most interns and residents, you will resist the temptation to find out. Your sense of duty and honor will command that you answer your page lest a patient lie in pain or die awaiting your call. However, if anecdotes help to reinforce the point, then here are two that were related to me. The first is told by an attending physician at a community hospital.

> We had this intern, Ken. He seemed to have trouble from the start. He went to a good medical school and had decent board scores. I was one of the faculty members that had interviewed him, and I had thought he would make a good resident. But somehow when he got here, he didn't seem as prepared as the other interns in his class. For their part, the other interns, and some of the senior residents, complained that Ken's patients were not well cared for and that they were constantly up late at night tying together his loose ends. On top of that, no one seemed to particularly like him. In the third month, I remember there was a formal complaint filed by one of the nurses. She said that Ken hadn't answered his pager. We talked to Ken and he swore that he never received the page. There was no adverse event because of the failed page, and we weren't sure whether the nurse just didn't like Ken. So we let it slide. In retrospect, we probably shouldn't have been so lenient the first time. A little while later, another nurse lodged a formal complaint. Again he denied it, but this time the complaint went into his permanent record in the department.
>
> Some of the other residents started coming forward to say that Ken was ignoring his pages on a fairly regular basis and they were being called to pick up his slack. One of the chief residents had a clever idea. He performed a sting operation.

The next time Ken was on call, the chief resident paged him to the floor. Ken didn't respond. The chief resident waited and paged again, and again. Ken didn't respond until the third page. Was he ever surprised when the chief resident picked up. Ken swore he hadn't received the first two pages. The chief resident then tested his pager with Ken standing in front of him and it worked just fine. The chief resident brought this information to us, and we suspended him at once.

On another note, this was the story of one intern who was working in a busy, urban hospital.

I was getting slammed. I was managing one chest pain and an older guy close to coding who had shortness of breath, and there were two patients who had fallen that I still had to see. My senior resident was on another floor dealing with something else. It was crazy. On top of all that, I had been paged three times for an orthopedic patient with hip pain. Orthopedics was full, and she had been dumped on us because she also had a history of an MI in the distant past. I gave her oxycodone, but they kept paging me. I wrote for another dose of oxycodone, and then one more when they paged again. When they kept paging from the ortho floor, I knew why they were paging and so I didn't answer it. I felt that she had been given enough narcotics and would just have to wait for a while because I had more critical patients to care for. Then, I got a call from my senior resident.

"Baker," my senior said. "Ortho floor has been paging you. Why haven't you answered?"

"It's that lady with hip pain." I told him matter-of-factly. "I'm managing a guy with chest pain, and I still have Mr. Johnson with shortness of breath. I gave her oxy. The medication might just need time to kick in. She'll be fine. I'll see her after."

127

"Baker," my resident's voice was crisp and quick to the point, "your hip pain lady has stopped breathing."

"What?" I asked, stopping breathing myself. "What are you talking about?"

"Don't worry. I told them to push Narcan. But go see her now."

I felt awful. I had overdosed her with narcs. Thank goodness my senior resident had answered the page. No matter what, from then on, I always answered.

 ## LESSON LEARNED

Nothing is more basic or important than being responsible and acting professionally. If you are on call, you need to answer your pager—no ifs, ands, or buts. The person paging you may have an unimportant or even trivial question for you. Then again, the person calling may need your help with someone with pain, shortness of breath, or something even more emergent. The patient may be dying. Regardless, it's your job to answer promptly, so do it.

GET SLEEP WHILE YOU CAN WHEN ON CALL

Don't stay awake while on call "just in case." This story was told to me by a colleague. I think it is very telling and a great example to learn from (rather than to have to experience first hand).

I had a very good senior resident. He was a foreign graduate and had actually been a surgeon in his home country. He seemed to know everything and was always extremely helpful to

128

the interns and other residents. In the middle of the year, I was very glad when I was placed on his ICU team for my first ICU rotation. The ICU was . . . well, the ICU. We had call every fourth night, and we'd sleep, oh, I'd say an hour or maybe, on a good night, two or three hours. No more than that. Still, at least we got some sleep. On my first call, we finished our work around four in the morning. Pre-rounds started before six, so while my resident went to sleep (or so I thought), I decided to stay up and start pre-rounding. I wanted to make a good impression on my ICU attending and the rest of the team.

I downed two cups of coffee and started writing my notes for rounds. I reviewed the labs and vitals, made notes of changes to medications, and got everything together. When rounds started at 6:30 AM, I hadn't slept a wink but felt good that I had stayed awake to prepare. That made my disappoint-ment more pointed when we started rounding. When I opened my mouth to present, I immediately noticed how tongue tied I had become. I couldn't make sense of anything. I presented labs for the wrong patient, gave updates on things that had occurred days ago, and generally made a mess of things. Rounds were a disaster. Luckily, my resident kept jumping in to save me. I learned my lesson that day. I need an hour, or at least 30 minutes of sleep to be able to function in the morning, especially when I'm tired at baseline (which pretty much every-one is in the ICU). Without a little cat nap, I become a bum-bling village idiot. With 30 minutes, I can make it through to after lunch. From then on, I made sure to get at least a little bit of sleep (when possible). This let me actually use the time productively when I was awake. My resident, I soon learned, wasn't doing the same.

My resident was excellent in so many ways. Like I said, he was always helping us out. Sometimes, though, particularly post-call, he seemed to forget everything. Only later, I would learn that he was going through a divorce and not sleeping much at home. In short, he was at the end of his rope, and the ICU, particularly the calls, were pushing him over the edge.

One morning, post-call, I noticed how tired he looked. "Didn't you sleep at all?" I asked.

"No, Tom, I don't sleep on call. I never do."

We were all tired, but he looked absolutely exhausted. "Can you function on so little sleep?"

"I'm used to it, Tom." He smiled. He always used my name when we spoke. "Tom, you know, I'm just very tired. I'm older than most of you guys. I just want to graduate and open up a little practice. But if I fall asleep at night, I'm worried I might miss something or not hear my pager. I don't want to do that."

I nodded. I understood because I was always worried about oversleeping my pager, too. But I was concerned for him. Through the course of the rotation, I watched as he continued to decompensate. Post-call, he gradually couldn't remember even basic information about patients. We made it through the rotation.

In the second half of the year, in a subsequent ICU rotation, one of his patients had a bad event. I didn't get the details but, less than five months before he should have graduated, he was suspended. I am certain it was because he was just so worn down and tired. I wished he would have slept a little during call. I think the bad event wouldn't have happened if he had just taken a little cat nap here and there. He was such a good physician. It was a real shame, and the administration did not stand up for him.

LESSON LEARNED

Some people can function on *no* sleep for a night or more. But, in my experience, more people *think* they can function on no sleep than actually can. I would strongly recommend that you allow yourself at least a little sleep, if possible, so that you can adequately use the time you *are* awake. I can get more done in an hour when I'm alert, with some sleep behind me, than in two hours in which I'm bone-tired and haven't slept. You'll find what works best for you. But, don't fool yourself into thinking you are able to get by on less sleep than you need just because you *wish* that were the case. Do yourself a favor and see things as they are. Take a nap if you can. Maybe you and your colleagues can work out covering each other while one gets a little rest. Getting even a little bit of sleep may just save you and your patient in the morning.

TAKE THE ELEVATOR IF IT'S AVAILABLE

Unless you are in extremely good shape, don't race up eight flights of stairs and then try running a code. This happened to me during internship—except I think it might have been six flights of stairs. In my hospital, as in most hospitals, when a code was called, the inpatient medicine teams *ran* to the code. That's the background for the following story.

An attending called out sick one day, and so three floor teams were rounding together with the same service attending. That made for a team of six interns, three residents, and four medical students. We had just met to start rounds on the first floor when a code was called on the 9th floor. The teams listened to the location, and then we ran to the elevator. The elevators could be notoriously slow in the morning. So, ten of us raced to the stairs and bounded up them.

At first, we were taking the stairs two at a time. Someone on the 9th floor was in cardiac arrest. We started slowing down around the 4th floor. By the 5th floor, most people were taking the steps one at a time. By the 6th floor, a couple of people paused to catch their breath. By the time we burst out of the stairwell onto the 9th floor, every one of us was huffing and puffing.

We looked ahead and saw the three interns who had waited for the elevator entering the patient's room where the code had been called. The rest of us crawled in after them, sweat glistening on our brows. I could feel my heart pounding, and I took a moment to lean against the wall. A crowd of residents from different teams had already arrived, anyway. I noticed that if I or the other interns who had taken the stairs had been asked to do chest compressions at that moment, we would have had a hard time as we were still trying to catch our breath.

It occurred to us, that if a life weren't expiring at that very moment, it would have been something of a comedy to see the lot of us young doctors—all sleep deprived, hungry, and tired—racing without thinking up so many stairs to leave us nearly useless when we were needed most.

LESSON LEARNED

I was in pretty good shape when I started internship, and we had a couple of runners on the team. However, between lack of sleep and a decreased amount of daily exercise, you too might find yourself less ready to climb several flights of stairs than you remember. The moral? Know yourself. My hat is off to firemen and other rescue workers who race up stairs with heavy packs on their backs. What they do is amazing. For us mortals who aren't in marathon condition, if there are more than a few flights between you and the code, consider taking the elevator (or perhaps have just one or two people take the stairs in case the elevator doesn't work).

👍 WEAR CLOTHING TO SLEEP IN THE CALL ROOM

Some people like to sleep naked. That's fine, just don't do it in the call room. A friend of mine in a residency program reported the following story to me.

A guy resident walked in on a girl intern sleeping naked in the call room. Needless to say, awkwardness ensued.

☝️ *LESSON LEARNED*

Those sheets might not look dirty, but you have to believe they aren't the cleanest. And your call room is not your home. Don't get too comfortable. Don't sleep in the nude.

👍 FIND AN UNOCCUPIED CALL ROOM IF POSSIBLE

The following was related to me by an intern at a community hospital. It is representative of a story I heard repeated by many interns. It only applies, however, to hospitals with more than one option for where an intern sleeps during call. Many hospitals have only one place, so the situation may be unavoidable.

It was my first call of the year. I finally made it into the call room around 3 AM. Our calls were arranged so that we had two interns on call, one intern who took night float, and one resident who supervised all three of us. The night float intern was busy in the ER all night doing admissions. The two call interns covered the floor. We had a call room in the basement and one on the 11th floor. Being the first night, my co-intern and I resolved to stay in the 11th floor call room together for moral as well as practical support. Yes, there were two beds. When I came back to the room, he was sleeping. I kicked off my shoes and fell into the other bed. No sooner had I started to drift to sleep than the pager went off. I flicked the light on and checked my pager but it wasn't me. I looked up to see Peter rubbing his eyes.

"It's me," he told me. "10th floor." He dialed. "On call returning a page . . . uh huh . . . uh huh . . ." Peter was still rubbing his eyes as he listened to the nurse on the other end of the line. "Okay, what was the pulse again? . . . I see." Peter covered the phone with one hand and asked me, "What do you give for a heart rate of 130 in a guy with COPD, short-ness of breath, and no chest pain?"

"You have to go see him," I told him.

A little while later, Peter returned. I woke up when he came into the room. Then I got a page. Throughout the rest of the night, we both discovered that when one of us finally got to sleep, the other would get a page. During a night when we could have possibly slept two or three hours, we ended up sleeping less than one, broken up by twice as many pages and phone calls. I learned my lesson pretty quickly, but I was sur-prised to see in the coming weeks and months how many people felt that they had to stay in the same room for continued "moral support." What does that mean? I thought they were insane. One night of moral support—okay, but for the whole year? Some of the interns even gave up on sleeping and just studied during the downtime or lounged on their beds, know-ing that one of the two of them would get a page soon enough.

LESSON LEARNED

My opinion here is that sleep is precious. If you can sleep on call, do sleep. Of course, there is a certain understated nobility to sharing the suffering. And, building camaraderie is a definite plus. But can't you bond over "war stories" from the floors in the morning or the next day? It's a balance, but just be aware of what you're setting yourself up for if you choose to stay in the same call room when you have an alternative. You're accepting less sleep and greater fatigue and thus poorer decision making in exchange for the comfort of having someone next to you to share your increased suffering. It's probably not the worst decision, but it's not one that I would recommend.

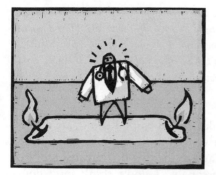

Chapter 7

Personal Survival and Well-Being: Do's and Don'ts

👍 AVOID DRIVING POST-CALL WHEN YOU'RE TOO TIRED

There is one incident that I will never forget.

I was post-call and had not slept all night. I was finishing my work and getting ready to go home. I lived in hospital-subsidized housing that was less than a block away from the hospital. I had been awake for over thirty hours and could not wait to get some sleep. One of the nurses saw me.

"Oh, you're still here, Dr. Cooper? I thought you had left. Are you going to drive home soon?"

*"Drive?" At the time I thought it was a ridiculous sugges-
tion. "I'm way too tired to drive right now. No, I live down the
block. It's just a short walk. I'm going home in a few minutes."
Drive? I couldn't drive after not sleeping 30 hours, right?
Would you? And yet, there I was writing prescriptions for my
patients.*

The hours they make interns work, I think, are an out-
rage. Even with the work-hour rules, I've seen many mistakes from interns and residents who were just too tired
to get it right. Personally, I don't think long hours
enhance doctor training. I think that hospital adminis-
trations want long resident hours so they can keep their
operational costs down. Many hospitals still don't
enforce the work hours because it is cheaper for them
not to and face whatever penalties might come their way
(usually none). It's the patients who suffer most because
of this. I remember being a third-year medical student
and watching an ob/gyn resident who hadn't slept in
more than 24 hours perform a new procedure for the
first time. Would you want an overworked, inexperienced
resident performing a procedure she had never done
before on you after she hadn't slept in more than a day?
Do you think that patient truly had informed consent?
Do you think the patient understood the condition of
the resident who was operating?

On an institutional level, the most egregious example
of lack of sleep I ever saw was during a pediatric rotation. The post-call intern had not slept all night, but she
was *required to stay* for the noon conference that lasted
from 12 to 1. So, dutifully, she stayed. Ironically, the
conference was a mandatory lecture that the hospital
required all residents to watch about the importance of

138

getting enough sleep. In the taped lecture we watched on the television set, we were told that the human body required a certain amount of sleep and that not getting enough impaired our judgment, dulled our senses, and had a variety of negative health consequences. The great irony was that the poor post-call intern kept dozing off during the lecture because she could barely keep her eyes open, but she wasn't allowed to go home and get some sleep until after the lecture!

Not everyone shares my opinion. Many doctors feel strongly that training while sleep deprived is essential to becoming a good doctor. After all, they argue, if you haven't learned to function as a doctor with little sleep, what will you do when a patient calls you in the middle of the night? I don't find this argument credible. But, this is a debate for another book.

✋ LESSON LEARNED

I have digressed and will now step off my work-hour rule soapbox and get back onto my hospital survival soapbox. The moral here is that you should not drive home after being on call if you are too tired. The risks of doing so are real, immediate, and extremely dangerous. In many residencies, interns have reported having had at least one car crash while attempting to drive home post-call. One internship class in particular was noted for all of their interns (except one) having had at least one minor car accident during the year.

When you are post-call, all you will want to do is go home. You'll be tired, feel dirty, and need a shower. You'll miss your bed and your significant other and/or your couch. You'll want the comforts that only home can give you. But if you're too tired, be honest with yourself and take a nap. Even an hour-long nap may give you the energy you need to drive home. I can't stress this one enough—don't drive if you are too tired. I know people who have fallen asleep behind the wheel and woken up only after their car crashed. It's not worth it. Interns and residents sometimes joke about it. Some wear their experiences like a badge of honor as if to say, "Look how hard core I am. I was so tired I fell asleep in my car while I was stopped at a traffic light. I was that tired!" That's not cool, and it's not honorable. It's stupid, dangerous, and irresponsible. Driving while exhausted will make you create more patients than you will have fixed by staying awake all night. Don't do it. Take a nap, use public transportation, walk, or have a friend drive you.

TRY NOT TO TAKE YOUR WORK HOME WITH YOU

This is a tough one. Presumably, you became a doctor at least in part because you care about other people. As an intern, you will see a lot of suffering. Personally, I think you should let your compassion show at work. I don't think it is healthy to block out emotions, as long as you continue to act professionally. But, as an intern, you will be spending a lot of time in the hospital— more than is healthy. So when you do leave the hospital doors and breathe fresh air, try your best to leave your work behind you. Don't worry—it will be right there waiting for you when you come back in a few hours. While you're at home, watching a movie, catching a nap, spending time with your significant other, enjoy those things. Enjoy your loved ones. I encourage you to share the events of your work day with your loved ones, but don't let your experiences at the hospital swallow you whole. Set your boundaries. You need down time when you can relax and feel good about relaxing.

> *A good friend of mine is one of the most caring persons I know. As an intern, she simply could not leave her work behind her. She dreamt about death nightly. She couldn't relax. It felt to her as though she couldn't breathe. She cried for each of the patients she couldn't make better. She never felt at ease at home because she knew her patients were still suffering. She was incredibly capable but barely made it through her internship because of this inability to compartmentalize and leave her work at the door.*

LESSON LEARNED

One of the oddities about internship is that after spending so much time at work, many people actually start to feel guilty when they do ultimately leave. They find it hard to relax even when they're home. They'll be cooking dinner and all of a sudden think, *"Oh my God, did I check the magnesium? . . . Oh, yes, I did."*

Do a good job at work and then leave it there. Patients don't want to see constant despair in their doctors. They want to see life, optimism, and inspiration. If you relax and enjoy life outside of work, you'll be a better doctor while at work.

TRY NOT TO TAKE YOUR PERSONAL LIFE TO WORK

This really isn't internship specific, but it is certainly applicable to internship. For many people, internship

141

is a time of great change. Relationships are stressed, finances may become strained as loans start coming due, and nerves are generally fried thanks to the pressure of your new job. Still, as best as you can, check your personal life at the door. You can talk about personal stuff with colleagues and friends at work. But, use common sense, and never burden your patients with your personal problems. As an example, consider the following story that took place at a large university hospital.

> *There was an intern who was going through a strain on her marriage during internship. Often, she started crying at work. She became short-tempered with her colleagues and patients. Her colleagues knew what was going on with her marriage, and they tried to be understanding, but ultimately she was told she had to change her ways or take a leave of absence from the program. She managed to cope and compartmentalize better, and she learned to be more professional at work, even while she was going through difficult times at home.*

LESSON LEARNED

The above is an extreme example of a mundane problem. We all have bad days. But when we come to work, and especially when we interact with patients, we have to check those bad days at the door. We have the responsibility of putting on our professional face when we see patients. That doesn't mean we have to be robots, far from it. But it does mean we have to have a professional manner. Think about always projecting calm, positive energy in everything you do. That's professionalism.

142

👍 ATTEND TO YOUR PERSONAL HYGIENE

This is one that hopefully you'll find obvious. Nevertheless, in the sleepless, stress-filled hours of internship, many have been known to forget. As an intern, you will sometimes go 24, 30, or even more hours straight without sleeping. During some rotations, particularly when you're on an ICU rotation, you'll be chronically tired. This is pretty much inevitable. When you get home, all you'll want to do is eat junk food, crash on the couch, and sleep. When you set your alarm for the morning, you will want to set it for as late as possible; snoozing once the alarm does go off to steal as many minutes of sleep as you can. Because of these demands on your time and energy, you will make sacrifices. You will go out to dinner less with your family and friends. You'll cut down on the number of movies you watch, stop exercising as much, and generally cut back or stop altogether the recreational things you most enjoy. You'll stop cooking and order out instead. And some of you will be tempted to stop maintaining proper hygiene—yes, even hygiene.

Most interns have felt the desire at some point to just roll out of bed, put on a pair of scrubs (dirty or clean—when you're that tired you stop caring), and show up to work. Sometimes, that means not shaving, showering, brushing hair and/or teeth, and generally keeping yourself groomed and professional. While most interns feel this impulse at some point, most also resist the impulse because of, well, because they do. But some don't resist it. Consider the following account

143

told to me by a resident who did her internship in a busy, urban hospital.

> We had an intern named Harold in our class who stopped taking care of himself for a while. In the beginning of the year, Harold seemed relatively well adjusted. Somewhere in the middle of the year, during his second ICU rotation, he started to change. He stopped shaving and rarely combed his hair. He would wear the same pair of scrubs every day. We all looked tired and overwhelmed in the ICU so at first we just teased him about his lack of grooming, but it kept getting worse. He started to have a certain unwashed smell. He didn't seem to be going crazy, he just seemed to not care about anything anymore. If anything, he seemed to be getting increasingly bitter and depressed. I tried talking to him but he would either just grunt or joke about it.
>
> Harold's behavior stopped being funny to the rest of us. Some of us were really worried about him. When he went back to the general medicine floors, we thought he would return to his old self. But he didn't. Not at first. He continued to wear scrubs constantly. When his attending finally told him to put on a tie, he did, but he wore the same tie, shirt, and pants constantly. In addition, his work in general continued to deteriorate. Mostly, it was the little things that he wasn't doing. He wouldn't record labs. He'd forget to sign out information.
>
> Finally, toward the end of the year he started coming out of it. He started bathing and dressing again. It was like watching him become human, again. His work improved, and by our third year of residency, we had pretty much forgotten about his internship slide. But, for a while, I can tell you that we weren't sure whether he was going to survive the program.

🤙 *LESSON LEARNED*

For those of you who may be more susceptible to forgetting about your cleanliness, don't do it, for the following reasons: First, self-respect. Second, you will feel better when you take the time to shower and make yourself presentable. There can be a feeling of losing a sense of yourself during difficult times of internship. Keeping to some very basic routines such as showering can help keep you grounded. Remember, this too shall pass. You'll get through internship. Try to do it with as much grace and cleanliness as possible.

👍 TRY THIS TECHNIQUE TO MAKE YOURSELF FEEL BETTER AND TO MAKE THE DAYS AND NIGHTS GO FASTER

A psychiatry resident gave a friend of mine a trick for getting through the long calls at the hospital. She told my friend to pretend that he was the star of his own television show about an intern in the hospital. I heard this story as a resident and used the game myself to make some of the longer calls pass by more quickly. Essentially, the "game" is to step outside yourself and watch yourself going through your day and night at the hospital. By doing this, all of a sudden, all of the small indignities of the hospital, all of the hardships and the annoyances take on a different, less consuming light.

Consider J.D., played by Zach Braff in *Scrubs* on NBC. J.D. probably doesn't enjoy being screamed at by Dr. Cox, and he certainly doesn't like being tormented by the janitor. But, for us *watching* J.D., it's hilarious.

In a similar way, your job at the hospital, using this game, is to step outside yourself. Watch yourself have to respond to a nurse calling you at 3 AM because a blood glucose was . . . oops, normal . . . never mind, doctor. It's not funny to you as you answer the phone . . . but it's funny as you *watch* yourself answer.

For any of you who have read Eckhart Tolle, this may sound very familiar. Tolle is a spiritual teacher and the author of the #1 *New York Times* bestseller *The Power of Now*. In his teachings, he talks about separating yourself from your mind. That is, he urges people to think of their minds as *tools,* and themselves as spiritual entities. In this way, a person can step outside of his or her mind and watch his or her thoughts. Of course, there is a commonality between Tolle and some eastern religions. But you don't have to be religious to use this tool.

Step outside yourself. Watch yourself going through your day as if you were the star of your own television show. You can make it a comedy or a drama. Hospitals are suited to both. Try playing a laugh track in your head when something preposterous happens—as it often does. The show also keeps you company as your colleagues go home and you're left alone in the hospital. It turns the clerks, nurses, residents from other services, and even patients into a colorful supporting cast for your lead. Truly, if your life as an intern does not make for a good sardonic humorous show, what does?

 PRESERVE YOUR DIGNITY

They can't take some things from you. They can take your time. They can take your sleep. They can work you like a dog and pay you peanuts. But there are things they can't take from you unless you give them away. When you're tired, exhausted, feeling dejected, like it will never end and you don't have reserves left in you, just remember, they can't take your dignity. That's yours to do with as you choose. Choose to keep it. In a million ways, they will try to make you doubt yourself and think less of yourself. Know who you are. Ground yourself in that self-confidence and never think less of yourself. The following story is from an intern in a small community hospital in Connecticut.

I spent a rotation during my internship in the emergency room. In general, the doctors there were terrific, caring individuals. There was one notable, ugly exception. He was an older guy who should have retired years ago or maybe just never should have become a physician in the first place. He treated the residents, and interns in particular, despicably. He berated us and told us we didn't know anything. He gave us meaningless tasks and then told us to stop wasting our time on them. I complained to my director, who told me that he knew about the attending but that there was nothing he could do about it. We, the other interns and I, would just have to deal with it. One time, this curmudgeon told me that one of the favorite aspects of his job was trying to destroy his residents' self-confidence. I asked him why. He shrugged.

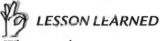

LESSON LEARNED

When people treat you poorly, let that reflect on them. You can't change others. You can change yourself, and you can mold your reactions to others, but don't spend your time trying to change someone else, particularly during internship. When I see an attending yelling, chastising a resident loudly for all the world to see in the middle of the hallway, I think it reflects badly on the attending. Keep your dignity and self-confidence with you. Display it with your body posture and speech. Display it quietly, confidently, and gracefully.

👍 MAINTAIN HEALTHY EATING HABITS

Resist the temptation to eat only fried food and junk food. We've all been there. We're tired, frustrated, and feeling drained, and so we reach for our comfort food of choice—pizza, candy, ice cream, milkshake, chicken fingers, cheeseburger. You know, comfort food. No matter what your job or position in life, you're going to have stress. There are a thousand and one self-help books about how to handle that stress without eating junk food. Suffice it to say, just be warned that when you're an intern, you will be dealing with stress on a daily basis for most days of the year. In addition, you will spend so much time in the hospital, that you won't have many outlets to relieve that stress even if you wanted to. Add to the above that foods available in most hospitals are not the healthiest by any stretch of the imagination, and you've got a perfect setup for a year of junk food. Consider the following account from an intern in a relatively large community hospital.

> The program director joked that, when he was an intern, the only joy he had all year was eating. He gained over 15 pounds from constantly eating cheeseburgers and junk food. He encouraged us to do the same to help keep our sanity. But

I didn't want to do that. The director was only in his late 40s and already had many health issues of his own.

✋ LESSON LEARNED

You probably know some people like the program director described above. Reaching for some comfort foods is probably inevitable. But there is a trend among interns, and residents in general, to comfort themselves with junk food and fried food daily. I urge you not to do this. Eating in an unhealthy manner is not without consequence. There are immediate health effects, such as swings in your energy and mood. And, there are potential long-term health consequences, even if you are relatively young and you only plan on eating unhealthy for the year. Bad habits are hard to break, and good ones are even harder to form. If you spend the year eating junk food, you may find it hard to stop when the year ends. Do your best to stay healthy despite the pressures. The healthier you eat, and the more time you find to exercise, the better you'll feel, and the better you'll be able to deal with the stress of the year.

Something that used to surprise me and now just disgusts me is how hospitals, *hospitals*, can peddle such unhealthy foods in their cafeterias. I guess you could call it capitalism at its best and worst. The only thing some hospital cafeterias are missing is a cigarette machine. Regardless of how you feel about them, they are a reality. You can almost always find some healthy foods, though. And you can always bring your own food from home. Just prepare it the night before. Your heart, arteries, liver, stomach, other organs, and state of mind will thank you.

149

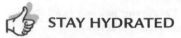 **STAY HYDRATED**

Keep a bottle of water with you and refill it often. Working as a doctor, and specifically as an intern, you will be on your feet for long hours. When you do happen to pause for nourishment, you may need to eat and drink quickly. Depending on your preference, you may end up drinking large quantities of coffee, tea, soda, and other caffeinated beverages that have a diuretic effect. Staying hydrated is not an easy intern task.

I remember talking with a physician who had just recovered from a kidney stone. He said that he believed doctors were at higher risk for stones because they are always talking to patients and moving from one room to the next, never pausing to keep themselves hydrated.

What are the benefits of staying hydrated? It will keep your risk of kidney stones down. It's also good for your heart, skin, muscles, and the rest of your body. Some people who are chronically mildly dehydrated (which in reality is probably most of the population) who increase their daily amount of fluid intake, and water in particular, report having more energy and feeling generally better.

Don't count on grabbing a drink here or there in the hospital. I would recommend getting a small bottle and filling it with water periodically over the course of the day. Try drinking the equivalent of at least eight glasses of water throughout the day. If you want a rough score card of how you're doing, look at your urine. If your urine is clear or pale yellow, you are probably taking in enough fluid. However, if you are drinking a lot of caffeinated drinks, your urine may be clear but your body still dehydrated. Drink lots of fluids and stay hydrated.

MAKE SURE THAT YOU ARE COVERED BY HEALTH INSURANCE

I dislike filling out almost any form. Thank goodness my wife helps me with those things now. But, whether or not you hate them, they are a necessary evil. Now that you are an intern, you are a working person. Some of you don't need this wake up call, others of you, and you know who you are, do. You need to worry now about things like paying off loans, paying rent, managing a budget, and making sure you are covered by health insurance. All of this means a lot of paperwork.

An intern at a large, respected university hospital filled out all of the appropriate papers to be covered by one of the hospital's health insurance policies. A few weeks into his residency, he received a letter saying that he hadn't in fact filled out one of the forms necessary for coverage. He called them and they said they would send the form. He never received the form, and he forgot about it. He figured he was covered because he noticed that the hospital was directly deducting health insurance payments from his paycheck. Later in the year, this intern got appendicitis. He ended up staying in the hospital for three days. To his surprise and utter frustration, his insurance company told him that the several thousand dollar bill was his to pay because he had never completed the paperwork for his health insurance. Naturally, the resident fought the insurance company.

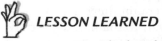

LESSON LEARNED

I am not certain whether the intern in the above story was ultimately reimbursed or not, but regardless, it was the source of a constant headache for several months.

It may be a pain if the papers don't go through right the first time, but make sure that you are covered by health insurance.

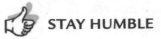 **STAY HUMBLE**

You're in a hospital, dealing with life and death on a daily basis. Nothing should inspire more humility in you. Don't get cocky or arrogant. Just remember that even once you know *a lot*, there remains even more that you still have to learn. Arrogance reveals itself in a million small ways throughout the day, making it very hard to hide. If you have arrogance in your heart, chances are that it will find a way to manifest itself even if you have the good sense to try and hide it. Remember your humility; internalize it.

> *"Don't you know by now, Jamie? You have to send the CBC in the purple top and the metabolic panel in the gold top. We've been here three months already."*
>
> *"Okay, thank you, Alex. I'm sorry, I just forgot. I sent it down wrong the first time and just didn't want to make the same mistake again."*

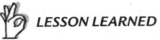 *LESSON LEARNED*

Alex may have picked things up more quickly than Jamie, but his arrogance will end up getting him into trouble at some point. We do learn a lot during internship. We learn so much that some of us start to think we know everything. Nothing could be farther from the truth. Your senior residents and your attendings are still learning, so how could you expect to know it all after only a few months, or even a couple of years, on the job? You will be learning from the first to the last day of internship, and that will just be the beginning of your learning. If you start to think you know everything, people will be less likely to help you—and then you'll really find out that you don't know as much as you had hoped. Just stay humble.

In internship, you see so much death and disease affecting so many people, some younger than you. I was told a story of a woman who had just finished her internal medicine residency and was getting ready to start a family and also a medical practice with her husband. Then, she was diagnosed with metastatic melanoma, and soon after she died. Remind yourself that you are going to walk out of that hospital at the end of the day and go to your warm home. If nothing else keeps you humble, it should be enough to consider your great fortune that you are healthy, loved, and able to care for others.

BE GIVING AND COMPASSIONATE

When I started medical school, the senior students put on a play for us. It was called *The Giving Tree* and was adapted from Shel Silverstein's children's book of the same name. I found this very amusing because my mother is a kindergarten teacher and at the end of every school year, her class puts on *The Giving Tree* play for the parents. For those of you who don't know, *The Giving Tree* is the story of a boy and a tree. When the boy is young, he plays in the tree's branches and the tree is happy. As he grows older, the boy has increasing demands on the tree. The tree loves the boy and wants to see him happy, so he tells the boy he can sell his apples for money. Later, the boy cuts the tree's branches to build a home, and then he cuts the trunk to build a boat. By the end of the story, the boy has become an old man, and the tree its only its stump left. The tree tells the old man to sit on its stump and rest. It is a beautiful story and you can interpret it in a variety of ways. My mother has her kindergartners put on the play to teach about giving. The tree always seems happy to help the boy. But the reason the senior medical students wanted to perform the play for us was to warn us to not be the tree.

The senior medical students wanted to advise us that we would have lots of demands on our time and energy. Patients would ask for as much as we could give and the seniors wanted to remind us to keep something for ourselves or we wouldn't have anything left to offer. They wanted us to pace ourselves through our careers. If we gave and gave and gave, they were afraid we would burn out and have nothing left for anyone, including ourselves. It is a point worth considering, especially as it seems to happen to some people.

I think you need to give as a person as well as a physician. In many ways, I disagree with the notion that giving something away means you have lost something. On the contrary, often when you give something away, you gain strength and energy from it. But, particularly during internship, you do have to be aware of the potential for burn out. Consider the following story told by an intern at a small, community hospital.

I was on call and had just gotten into bed. It must have been close to 4 AM. I was exhausted. The nurse called me for a patient on Green 7 whose Percocet order had expired. I tried

154

to give her a verbal order but she said she needed it written. I told her I was in the middle of something but would be there soon. Green 7 was all the way across the hospital. I was so tired and I knew that if I went there then, I wouldn't get any sleep at all. I needed at least 30 minutes that night or I'd be dead the next day. So I figured the patient could live for 30 minutes with the pain or maybe have a Tylenol until I got there. I mean, it was the other resident's fault for letting the order expire, you know? And, why couldn't that nurse just take my verbal order? She could have found some pain meds to give. She was just trying to give me a hard time. So I took a short cat-nap and went to write the order afterward.

LESSON LEARNED

This, too, happens all too often. You get so tired, and it becomes easy to forget what you are doing and why you are there in the first place. Imagine that the patient lying on Green 7 were your mother. Would you let her lie for 30 minutes in agony while you napped? Being an intern is tough work. You see so much pain, suffering, and dying that it can become routine. If a patient isn't crashing, you start to think their needs are not so important. You think that since pain won't kill the patient, it's not a priority. Believe me, for that patient, pain is most certainly a priority. It should be for you as well. Sometimes, if you are dealing with a patient who really is crashing, you have to prioritize. You can't run and write for pain medications if you are doing chest compressions, for example. But when the code is over or when you've finished giving IV Lopressor to break someone out of a-fib, then go over and write for the pain medications. Don't lose your compassion.

Consider the following story told by another intern at the same hospital.

I was done for the day and looking forward to going home to see my wife. I remembered that Mr. X's wife had wanted to talk to me at some point. I remember her well. She was one of those people who was very kind but who could talk for a long, long time. I thought about putting off the conversation. After all, my attending or resident should have been the one to talk to her. They knew more than I did about how her husband was doing. I was tired. I longed for my wife and for dinner. But I got along well with Mr. X's wife, and she wanted to talk.

I went to the room and sat with Mr. X and his wife. Twenty minutes later, Mr. X's wife said, "Thank you," her eyes glistening. "Thank you for sitting and explaining all of this. I know it's late." I smiled and held her hand. "Anytime," I told her. "It's my pleasure." And, I realized, somewhat surprised, it was.

I didn't leave the hospital feeling twenty minutes more tired. I felt alive and energized for the first time in weeks. The buzz lasted into the next day when I actually looked forward to coming back to work.

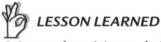 **LESSON LEARNED**

It is true that giving and giving more can sometimes leave you feeling somewhat drained. That is one of the reasons that it is so important to maintain relationships and activities you enjoy outside of work. Also, remember why you went into medicine, and what a unique opportunity you have to actually help people. Sometimes, the extra mile ends up giving you more fuel, not costing you. Yes, it may cost you time, but it will likely pay you back richly with good energy. I urge you—don't lose your compassion. Your compassion is, in many ways, your link to your humanity.

👍 WRITE PRESCRIPTIONS FOR PATIENTS ONLY

Don't trade pain killer prescriptions for marijuana in the parking lot of the clinic (I'm not making this stuff up). I don't think you really need this piece of advice. But, I know of at least *one* person who could have used this advice prior to his family practice residency. If he had read *and followed* it, it would have saved him several court dates and a lot of trouble and embarrassment, not to mention his job. I offer this true story to remind you that, once in a while, doctors do terrible, incredibly stupid things, and they get caught. Don't be one of these guys.

It was in the back of a clinic that sat in a small city on a street that roughly marked the boundary between the rich and poor neighborhoods. A resident sauntered into a dimly lit parking lot after clinic. There, he met a man dressed in street clothes.

"Who do I make the prescription out to?" James asked. "John Jackson," said the man in street clothes. "Make it for Percocet. Give me 120 pills."

James didn't ask if John Jackson was in fact the man's name or if he was actually in pain. He knew the answer to at least the latter was probably "no." James wrote out the prescription and handed it over to "Mr. Jackson" anyway, expecting to receive a bag of marijuana in exchange. What James didn't know was that Mr. Jackson was an undercover police officer, and James' life would never be quite the same.

LESSON LEARNED

It happens. I'd be surprised if there aren't plenty more stories like that one. There are good and bad people who become doctors just as there are in every other profession. Anyway, obviously don't do it, and tell the appropriate law enforcement agency and the appropriate person in your hospital if you hear of someone else doing it.

GET YOURSELF A GOOD PAIR OF COMFORTABLE SHOES

Maybe this is the most important piece of advice. Shoes, comfortable shoes. You already know how important comfortable shoes are from medical school rotations. Well, it only gets harder on your feet during internship. For one, your feet are getting older. Two, your hours are getting longer. When it comes to your footwear, this is not the time to pinch pennies. Do yourself a favor and get a good a pair of comfortable shoes.

TAKE PRIDE IN WHAT YOU DO

You're a doctor, for crying out loud. Of course you should take pride in what you do. Yet, many of us don't. We get tired, beaten down from long hours, a perceived lack of respect from those around us, low pay, and what we perceive as patients who sometimes take our efforts for granted. Nonsense. Don't let that stuff get to you.

158

We work long hours, but we have a lot of responsibility. Patients might seem less than grateful sometimes, but they're probably more scared and frustrated with their situation than anything else. Attendings, residents, and nurses might abuse us from time to time, but they usually want the best from us and are trying to push us to achieve it or they have their own issues. Either way, don't let it get to you. Hold your pride inside yourself and be sure to display it with grace and humility in everything you do.

👍 MAKE SURE THAT THERE IS A LOCK ON YOUR CALL ROOM DOOR

If you think that because you are a doctor, or because you are working in a hospital, that you don't have to worry about your personal safety, please wake up. Of course, some hospitals are safer than others. You can use your common sense in this regard. However, though not common, there *are* stories of interns and residents being attacked and raped while on call at the hospital.

Please, do make sure there is a lock on your call room door. This applies more to women, but guys should also be aware. Also, be aware of your surroundings, particularly late at night. Dark, empty staircases are not good places to go. Hospitals are typically not in the best parts of town. You may be safer than you are outside on the street, but you are not "safe." The minimum you can do is make sure there is a lock on the call room door. If there isn't one, demand that one be placed immediately.

A final word on safety. Especially at the beginning of the year, you don't really know your coworkers. There is at least one report of a resident raping an intern. The hospital, not wanting the bad publicity, apparently did everything it could to keep the story out of the papers. I'm not trying to make anyone paranoid, but you do have to remember that there are bad people around you in a hospital, just as in the rest of life, so don't let your guard down.

VENT WHEN YOU NEED TO, BUT NOT WHEN YOU DON'T

There is a lot to complain about during internship. A lot. You have your pick: Crashing patients, feeling like you don't know anything after you've been studying for more than the past 20 years of your life, attendings who don't appreciate you, residents who forgot what it is like to be an intern, crappy food, long hours, vomit, blood, feces, and urine that gets on your white coat, sundowning patients who take a swing at you—if you like to complain, you've hit the jackpot.

There is a lot of good in complaining. As I mentioned in the beginning of this book, some of my favorite times in residency have been spent shooting the breeze, swapping stories, and complaining about the status quo with fellow residents and interns "in the trenches" with me. It's a good bonding experience between you and your colleagues to have a satisfying "bitch session" every once in a while. This is especially true if the bitching is good-natured. But, you have to have limits. The material is so rich, so promising, that if you're not careful, you may spend all of your time complaining, as the stories are endless. But that's not healthy.

Many interns and residents have ample reason for their griping, but they let all of their energy get eaten

up by the circumstances and their subsequent persever-
ation on those circumstances. You have to be able to
step away from the madness or it will suck you in and
swallow you whole. Know when enough is enough.

> *To take this to an extreme, you can imagine two colleagues*
> *going out for a drink after work and consoling each other about*
> *their day. There's nothing wrong with that. They may go*
> *through a beer or two, or even three, and talk about their*
> *attending who keeps riding them, their patients (no names—*
> *HIPAA forbids it, so take it seriously) who tried to bite them*
> *and then threw up on their shoes, and the cafeteria food that*
> *gave two of their colleagues heartburn and made another one*
> *sick. They may even discuss the cockroaches in the call room.*
> *But if those two guys are still at the bar four hours later, on*
> *their eighth beer, still complaining, it's gone too far. Find some-*
> *thing else to talk about. Let yourself get out of the hospital*
> *when you're not there.*

LESSON LEARNED

As the Buddha teaches: pain is inevitable, suffering is
optional. Try to keep your suffering to a minimum.
Not dwelling on your complaints (valid as they may be)
for too long will help.

WASH YOUR HANDS FREQUENTLY—VERY FREQUENTLY WHEN SEEING PATIENTS

In 1847, a Hungarian physician, Ignaz Semmelweis, discovered that when doctors washed their hands with an
antiseptic solution, they reduced the infant mortality

rate drastically (from more than 12% to less than 3%). Only decades later, when Pasteur and others conducted experiments that clearly demonstrated the germ theory, would most of Europe come to accept the theory. Today, we know that hand washing reduces the chance of nosocomial infection, and it also reduces the physicians' chances of catching infections from their patients. Why, then, do so many of us still not wash our hands?

You wash your hands, of course. Or, do you? Consider that in one hospital in Australia, doctors self-reported hand washing 73% of the time, while their observed hospital rate was a paltry 9%!

In Cedar-Sinai Hospital in Los Angeles, compliance was found to be about 65%. After a series of initiatives, including handing out free Starbucks coupons for hand washing, compliance rose to 80%. Cedar-Sinai Hospital was not satisfied with this figure and finally figured out a way to convince its physicians to wash their hands. After a lunch meeting of top doctors in the hospital, the hospital's epidemiologist pressed the hands of the doctors into Petri dishes for culture. What grew on the dishes was photographed. The photographs were so vivid that the administration turned the picture of one of the hands covered with bacterial colonies into the hospital screensaver. Once word got out about the "experiment" and the screensaver was seen, hospital compliance for hand washing rose to close to 100%.

✌️ *LESSON LEARNED*

Do wash your hands. Wash your hands before you see a patient and after you see the patient. Wash them periodically during the day and before you eat. Most hospitals now have Purell or other waterless hand sanitizer on the walls. Use them. Wash your hands for at least 15 seconds or roughly the time it takes you to sing "Happy Birthday" to yourself (or aloud if you so choose). And, when you get home, wash your hands again. This practice will help keep your patients, you, and your family healthier.

👍 ENJOY THE LITTLE THINGS

Remember to take moments for yourself. The following account comes from a community hospital:

Sunday morning, early: My second Saturday night call on this new service, and it was just like the first: Two codes and neither made it. One heart failure patient had an exacerbation and we sent him to the unit. One patient with COPD needed close monitoring. Two other patients were ruled out for MI. We admitted four new patients to the floor. This month, I could tell, was going to be a long one.

It wasn't so much that I had had a bad night. It was that I knew I was going to be there for another four or five hours and then would have to return Monday morning and start the whole thing again. I checked my watch. 5:28 AM. I stretched and yawned and took a sip of my coffee. It was still hot and burned as it went down. I looked down at the change the cashier had placed in front of me. I forced a smile. "Thanks," I said and put the coins into my white coat.

I could hear the coins jingle as I made my way slowly to the elevator. In the elevator, I heard the all-too-familiar "Beep, Beep." I looked down. It was the 8th floor calling, again. I had been heading to the 3rd floor to check on the

163

COPD patient, but I took the elevator straight to the 8th, wondering what was in store for me now. Besides the stop at the 3rd floor, the elevator went directly to eight. It would be another hour and a half before the elevator would get busy.

The elevator doors opened and I turned the corner. I stopped, coffee in hand. There was a large window down the hall. I passed by it all day long. This time I walked up to it. The glass was cold to touch. My hospital was only eleven floors high, but it was by far the tallest building around. Being from the city, sometimes the location made me feel isolated. But at that moment, I felt different. Autumn had started and the trees were changing colors. Through the cold glass, a tapestry of yellow, gold, and orange rolled into the horizon, dotted by small clusters of houses.

I watched a lone car winding its way through the streets. It was small and blue. It intermittently disappeared beneath the trees. I wondered where the driver was headed and was heartened to remember that there was life outside the hospital after all. I watched a bird soaring in the sky.

"Beep, beep." I looked down. It was the 8th floor again. I took another sip of my coffee. I knew I had to go. With the image of the trees and the world outside in my mind, I turned my back to the glass and headed down the hall. This time, however, I had a renewed sense of energy. I couldn't articulate exactly why, but I felt, in some small way, revitalized.

LESSON LEARNED

Our days are made up of a billion small moments. Most of these moments will be spent doing things for other people. Do take a few moments for yourself and enjoy the little things. These are the moments that will matter. Take small moments, capture your feelings, watch them, enjoy them for what they are, realize that for all your triumphs and tribulations, your place in the universe is truly small. Enjoy that, too.

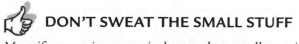 **DON'T SWEAT THE SMALL STUFF**

My wife sometimes reminds me that small worries make small people. On a daily basis in the hospital, you will likely suffer at least some small indignities. People will be rude, ungrateful, inappropriate, bump into you, ask you to hurry up, tell you to slow down, be disrespectful, be condescending, and/or put you out in some way. This doesn't necessarily reflect on you. This is just the way that hospitals and its inhabitants are. It's the way life is. Try to keep perspective. Stay above the fray.

You'll hear it all day long.

"Then he said that I had to check the metabolic panel. Why do I have to do that? Shouldn't that be Sandeep's job?"

"She asked me to switch the Thursday call but doesn't she know that Thursday call is better than Wednesday? Why should I have to make that switch?"

"Why can't the nurse just give the insulin? Why does she call me about that?"

"If that patient's wife asks to speak to me one more time, I'm going to scream. Doesn't she realize how busy I am? I don't know why her husband's insurance is denying the nursing home he wants. Why can't the social worker deal with it?"

And so on.

LESSON LEARNED

Keep sight of the big picture. Ask yourself if something is really worth your angst. You only have a given amount of energy, so use it wisely. If you spend it obsessing over why your attending is making you stay late again, you'll have less energy when you do get home to enjoy, and I mean really enjoy, the good stuff. Don't sweat the small stuff.

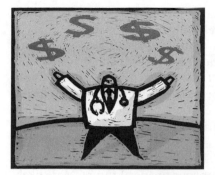

Chapter 8

Financial and Career Planning: Do's and Don'ts

👍 GIVE SERIOUS CONSIDERATION TO YOUR FUTURE FINANCES

Think about starting a 401K, 403b, IRA, Roth IRA, or other financial savings plan as an intern. As an intern, you won't make very much money compared with your future earning potential. In addition, you will have significant expenses such as rent, food, housing, and loan repayments, not to mention a little entertainment! Sometimes, it can feel like you are just squeaking by financially. This is not a "get rich quick" piece of advice and this is not a "financial help" book. There are plenty of those out there. Still, no matter how tight you may

167

feel your finances are, I encourage you to at least think about doing yourself a big favor by starting a financial plan sooner rather than later. I have learned that it is never too soon. Your hospital will almost surely have something like a 401K or 403b. You may also be able to open a Roth IRA or an IRA. Again, this isn't an investment book, but give serious consideration to making it a point to talk to a financial planner as early as possible in residency.

No one is going to go out of their way at your hospital to talk to you about your financial future. More likely, they'll just quip, "Don't worry, you'll make plenty later." That's true. But just as your income will greatly increase, so will your expenses. Start saving now. Even just a thousand dollars wisely invested today may add up to a significant amount by the time you are looking to retire. As much as possible, make it a habit to save a percentage of your earnings through pretax savings. That is essentially what a 401K, 403b, and IRA do. They're a way for you to save and invest money for your retirement without having to pay income tax on it.

In medical school, we really don't get enough financial education, if any. If you don't educate yourself, no one will do it for you. The sky won't fall if you fail to educate yourself, but on the flipside, if you *do* get ahead of the curve and start investing wisely, with professional help, now, I think you will thank yourself later.

A few people who have read earlier drafts of this book have asked me for specific recommendations about 401K, 403b, how much to save, IRAs, Roth IRAs, and so forth. I hesitate to provide specific advice here because everyone's situation is different, and in any case, I'm not the most qualified person to give specific advice. I'm a physician like you, after all, and not a financial planner. What I do feel confident saying is that you should make it a priority, *a high priority,* to speak with a financial advisor. Ideally, if you ask around, you should be able to find someone with a good reputation. If not, your hospital should be able to put you in touch with one. Just make sure that you are talking to someone that you feel comfortable with and who has experience.

Also, consider consolidating your loans and then *not* paying them off immediately. Think about investing that money instead if the interest rates are right. There are various factors that you should consider when deciding if and *when* you should consolidate, but often consolidation can get you a lower interest rate. You should talk to a financial planner or accountant you trust about all your options regarding consolidation.

Part of your conversation with your financial advisor should include the possibility of *not* paying your loan off right away. The reason to consider postponing paying back your loans is because you may be able to make a safe investment that pays you back more interest than your consolidated loan is costing you. For example, at the end of medical school, my consolidated loan interest rate was approximately 3%. During internship, rather than paying off the loan right away, I invested in a CD that was earning approximately 6% interest. This strategy won't make you rich, but if you can net yourself a few extra hundred or thousand dollars by doing it, why wouldn't you?

The above scenario may not fit your economic situation, which is why discussion with a financial advisor or accountant is worth the investment of your time. You may decide that consolidation is not in your best interest, and that paying off your loan immediately makes most sense for you, but at least you will have explored all of your options.

👍 LEARN TO WORK OUTSIDE YOUR COMFORT ZONE

Don't only do what is comfortable. There are two important reasons to broaden your set of skills. First, if you are always afraid of doing, say, an ABG (which is actually quite easy once you've done a few) then you will always be worried, wondering—what if I have to do an ABG on this patient? When you get called in the middle of the night to evaluate a patient, in the back of your mind will be the doubt—*what do I do if I need to get an ABG?* As a result, you'll not only try to convince yourself that an ABG is not necessary even when it might be, but you'll have the added noise of back-ground anxiety as well. You have enough anxiety as an intern without adding to it the fear of going outside your comfort zone.

The other important reason to do something that is not most comfortable is because there is a hospital Murphy's Law: If you are afraid of doing blood draws, you'll have blood draws to do. If you are unsure how to manage a patient with renal failure and thus try to dump all such patients on another team, you will end up with a team full of renal failure patients. If you run from it, sure as death and taxes, it will find you. So run to it, and conquer it with bravado. The following account is from a friend and colleague at a community hospital.

170

I liked outpatient clinic. It took place every Wednesday. We'd see everything there. It was a nice change of pace from the wards. Having said that, I hated, and I mean hated doing gynecology exams. They weren't a frequent occurrence in the clinic, but every couple of weeks, we'd have one or two. For the first couple of months, I'd look over the schedule and see their chief complaints and try to trade patients to avoid the ones I thought might need a gyn exam. Usually I was successful, but once in a while I wasn't. Part of the problem, I came to realize, was that I just hadn't done enough gyn exams during medical school to feel comfortable doing them. My inexperience made me fumble more and feel more self-conscious, making the whole process even more uncomfortable. The attending always had to repeat my exam anyway, making me feel like I was wasting everyone's time and just putting the woman through unnecessary discomfort.

What was worse still was that I slowly started to not look forward to the clinic, and I realized the reason why was simply that I dreaded the possibility of a gyn exam. The longer I went without feeling confident doing a gyn exam, the more I felt I should know and so couldn't ask. I hated not looking forward to the one part of internship that I actually used to like, but I couldn't help it. I told one of my seniors and he gave me advice that changed the rest of my year.

He said to me, "Don't just stop avoiding the gyn exams. Seek them out. Do as many as you can. Ask your attending to help you.

"Think of yourself as a soldier charging up a hill. If you charge up slowly, tentatively, then you won't make any progress, and the enemy will cut you down in short order. But if you charge up the hill at a sprint, you may get some shrapnel in your limbs, but you'll make it to the top. And once you're at the top, you'll take control of the situation and won't have to always be in fear."

I took my senior's advice. I charged up the hill, hating every minute of it. But after doing several exams with this new mindset, I shed my fears. The whole experience became much easier, and I began to enjoy the clinic again.

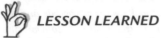

LESSON LEARNED

While the intern in the above story had trouble with gynecology exams and had to overcome his inhibitions by doing as many as possible, the same is true for doing blood draws, EKGs, ABGs, central lines, and taking complex histories, for example. You know what you don't feel comfortable with. If you don't know something and feel yourself pulling back from it, it is always best to dive in and take control of it. Ask as many questions as you can, understand that it may be awkward at first but that it will get better. If there is a procedure you dread, get someone to supervise you as needed and do it again and again. You and your patients will be better off for your determined charge up the hill.

REMEMBER THAT FUN DOES NOT ALWAYS EQUAL HAPPINESS

Everyone has different ideas of what is fun. Sure, we all tend to agree on some. During internship, you'll be doing less of those things. But that doesn't mean that you can't be happy. Quite the contrary. You're a doctor and you're becoming an experienced one.

When I was contemplating applying for a fellowship, a very good friend who was a few years ahead of me and had already done his fellowship gave me some excellent advice. He said, "Just remember, while you're doing the fellowship, if you decide to do it, that you *wanted* to do it." In other words, he was saying that it was going to be a hard year, and I was going to have to work very hard, but that if I remembered that I had chosen it, and how much I wanted it, then the work would be a lot easier to deal with. This is terrific advice for surviving internship as well. Now, when I have friends going through internship or residency or fellowship, I give them the same advice.

When you're spending those long hours as an intern, try to remember how much you wanted to be there. Remember how much you wanted to get into medical school and how proud you and your family were! Remember how much you wanted to get your internship and residency and how much you were looking forward to becoming an attending physician and having your own practice. Well, you're on your way! You're doing it! Sure, the novelty of being a "doctor" wears thin pretty quickly. But remember how much you looked forward to that. Hold on to that feeling and it will help sustain you.

You may or may not find that putting in IVs, drawing blood, doing ABGs, placing central lines, making high-pressured decisions, writing notes, etc., is "fun." But whether or not you have fun doing all of these things doesn't necessarily affect how happy you are or should be. People sometimes get into trouble by using fun as a yardstick to measure their happiness. They think, "Well, I'm at the park and it's a nice day, so I'm happy." Or, they think, "I'm stuck in the hospital and it's sunny outside. All my friends are at the beach . . . and I am miserable." Happiness is a reflection of your inner satisfaction and how you interpret the events around you. A prize fighter training for a big fight may not be having fun when he (or she) is doing his 300th sit-up, but there's no place he'd rather be and nothing he'd rather be doing. And, there is no time when he's likely to be happier. Having a purpose, a mission that you find worthwhile and good, and actively pursuing the fulfillment of that mission makes for some of the happiest people.

START THINKING ABOUT WHAT YOU WANT TO DO AFTER RESIDENCY, AND PLAN ACCORDINGLY

My father once told me a story about his investment broker that I have always remembered. My father's investment broker said to him, "You know, I will look after your money. These are the investments that I am recommending. But you should keep watch of your money, too. No one will ever take as good care of your money as you, because it's *your* money." Sometimes I tell this story to my patients. I tell them, "These are the steps that I am recommending for you to make yourself healthy. But, in the end, it's *your* body and it's your choice. I can give you this injection and make you feel better . . . but at the end of the day, no one can or will take as good care of your body as you can. It's *your* body."

No one can safeguard your money or your health as much as you can. And no one will look after your career as much as you can. It's *your* career, and you have to look after it and take responsibility for it.

174

In high school, people around you would probably have prodded you along to college if you hadn't been self-motivated. In college, you may have had counselors to make sure you had direction. Once you showed interest in medicine, they probably directed you to the premedical office. Even in medical school, your dean or various mentors may have prodded you along to a given residency. Those days are over. If you are interested in doing a fellowship or obtaining a certain specialization or expertise that is at all competitive, the time to start thinking about it is yesterday—or at least today.

This is not to say that you need to know what you want to do after residency. You don't, and, in fact, most people don't know when they're interns. Or, they think they do, but they will change their mind. If you think you know, my advice to you is to start preparing yourself for it now. Furthermore, even if you don't think you know, I would advise you to do what you can to keep your options open.

What does this mean? How do you plan for fellowship as an intern? How do you "keep your options open"? For starters, it means keeping your eyes open. Read about the different specialties. When possible, spend time with the specialists. Every field, every specialty is different. They all will look for slightly different things. But, in general, doing research is a strong plus for any field. Get involved with a research project early. It doesn't have to be a double-blind, placebo-controlled study. Start with a case report. Or perhaps a retrospective analysis. If you announce that you are interested in research, and if you show that you are willing to do the leg work for a study or case report, you will be surprised at how many attendings will come to you with their projects. I suggest that you start off small. Don't bite off a large project that doesn't have IRB approval and might not ever happen. Or, if you do that, *also* do something that you can get done in a reasonable amount of time, such as a case report. But, regardless of what research project you do, get involved.

LESSON LEARNED

The take-home point for this section is don't wait for the specialist to come to you and ask if you're interested in what they do. *Be aggressive and enthusiastic.* Go to the specialist.

REMEMBER THE GENERIC NAMES OF MEDICATIONS

As a medical student, you are still fairly close to your pharmacology studies. You still are used to using generic names for medications. In fact, when I was a student, I knew the names for the generic medications, but often didn't know the trade names. As an intern, this knowledge base begins to flip, and it flips quickly. You get used to speaking in terms of trade names. You write prescriptions for trade-name drugs. Often, many interns soon begin forgetting the generic names. Don't let this happen. Make a point of remembering both the generic and the trade names. It is a lot harder to go back and relearn the generic names than it is to simply never forget them in the first place.

When you talk of "Paxil" remember that you are really talking about paroxetine, an SSRI. Remembering this will help you remember what class of medication the drug is, the side effects, indications, etc. It will help you think of alternative medications in the event that an insurance company does not cover the particular trade-name drug. It will also help you when you take your Step III and specialty board examinations, because those tests are more likely to ask you about furosemide instead of "Lasix."

BE AWARE THAT YOU ARE STARTING A LEARNING PROCESS IN INTERNSHIP AND RESIDENCY, NOT COMPLETING ONE

I heard an associate professor of surgery speak at a conference. He had completed a fellowship at Harvard in spinal surgery 12 years prior. He noted that 60 to 70% of what he did in his current practice involved procedures he had *not* learned in residency or fellowship. His point, of course, was not in the least to imply that he had inadequate training. Rather, he was highlighting the ever-changing nature of medicine.

What you learn in your years of training is critical. It forms the backbone and first layer of meat of your medical knowledge. Onto this base, you will slowly add bulk and nuance during your years of practice. Thus it is important that you not only learn a large volume of information during training, but that you also learn *how* to learn quickly.

Understand concepts and frameworks. If you memorize a treatment but not *why* the treatment is done, then when innovations emerge, you won't understand why they are considered to potentially be effective or how to evaluate them. If you do understand the concepts, you'll be able to critically evaluate them better and maybe make some new discoveries of your own.

👍 READ AND RESEARCH EVEN THOUGH IT'S TEMPTING NOT TO

As I was putting this book together, I spoke to several interns who were just finishing their intern year. One of the interns said something that struck a chord with me. She said, "I tried reading at the beginning of the year. I read about all my patients, you know? If they had heart failure, I read about heart failure and looked up recent articles about current treatments. If they were going for an angioplasty, I read about angioplasty. I'd get home bone tired but would force myself to sit and study for a couple of hours before going to sleep. That lasted all of, I don't know, three weeks. Then I realized it just wasn't worth it. I learned that the hard way. Don't read your first year. Just survive it! I think you'll have plenty of time to read later. Tell them that."

I talked to many other people on this point, trying to arrive at a consensus. Should interns spend their precious time reading during internship? Or, should they just put their heads down, learn what they need to do to survive, plow ahead, and worry about reading later? There was no consensus to be found. Most people did *not* spend a great deal of time reading during internship, but some wished they had. A few echoed my own experience. I heard the following from one senior resident who reflected back on his internship year.

I didn't think about reading much in the beginning. There were so many other things to figure out. Like, where is the call room? What is the combination for the call room? How do I use the computers? How do I dictate a D/C summary?

178

Which patients are service, and which are private, and what are my responsibilities for both? How do I order a CBC and BMP? Does that include magnesium or is that a separate order?

Once I got home, I was so tired I just wanted to fall into bed. So, reading wasn't high on my list for the first month or two. But, gradually, as I began to understand why we were ordering various tests, I began to be more comfortable in the hospital. I started to ask more questions and wanted to know more. So I would go home or grab a few minutes here and there in the hospital and read about a condition that one of my patients had. Even just a little reading was interesting. I wouldn't spend more than a half hour a day or night reading outside of what I had to, but I'd read just enough to make things in the hospital clearer. Soon, I realized that there were some days I didn't want to read . . . but, if I forced myself to read on those days, just a little, then slowly but surely I began to feel much more like a doctor and not just a guy in a white coat trying to keep his head above water.

LESSON LEARNED

My own experience was similar to the above account. When I started, I had a demanding and good senior who was always asking me questions and forcing me to think. Instead of just blindly ordering labs and recording the results, she pushed me to understand why each thing was being done. It wasn't highly intellectual work, but if you don't give it at least some thought, then you find yourself becoming a highly efficient assistant to your resident and attending but not truly absorbing all that is going on around and in front of

179

you. Once I understood *why* things were being done, *why* a lab was ordered or not ordered, or *why* a patient was sent for this or that test, then I began to enjoy the process more. I also started reading, slowly, for myself. I'd read no more than an hour a day, and usually it was more like 15 minutes. I would read just enough so that at the end of the day, I could say that I taught myself at least one new thing. One good time to read, I found, was during the few minutes of down time during the day. I carried a book in my pocket and would make sure I had read a small section by the end of the day. I think that is a good habit to get into.

The mistake, I think, that some people get into is to try and read *too* much each day. They seem to feel that if they are not reading and understanding a whole chapter of a textbook or a couple of articles, it's not worth doing. This process, I feel, is too rigorous to maintain for an entire year of internship. Internship demands too much of your time and energy. Besides, who wants to spend *all* of their time outside the hospital studying? Instead, I recommend a gentler approach.

Read here. Read there. If there is a boring lunchtime lecture that you know you are going to be day dreaming through, bring an article and keep it on the table in front of you. Respectfully (meaning not obviously) glance through it while you're eating. When you are waiting for your senior resident or attending, read a paragraph. Learn the presenting symptoms of pancreatitis or how to manage diabetic ketoacidosis. Ideally, read a paragraph about a pathology of one of the patients on your service. When you try later to recall aspects of the pathology, it will be easier to remember the characteristics, symptoms, and findings that your patient had rather than an abstract case out of your textbook.

In sum, I think there are three main reasons to start reading a little at a time during internship. First and foremost, it will help you understand your patients and how to help them. This will make the process much more enjoyable for you. It will give you a sense (real or not) of some control in the hospital. This will diminish your anxiety and give you a feeling of empowerment. If you know what is going on and what to look for, you can ask the right questions and help direct care. If you don't, you will feel more and more lost.

Second, it's a very good habit to develop. It's hard to discipline yourself to read all the time. It gets easier as you become more senior in the process, because you have more time and because you can read more about specialized topics that may interest you—but it's never easy. Residency is almost always going to demand a lot of your time and energy, as will being an attending. Life responsibilities (e.g., family) will likely only increase, not decrease. All of these evolutions are good things, but the sooner you get in the habit of reading a little each day, the sooner you will think of it as you think of brushing your teeth. You wouldn't go to bed without brushing your teeth (if you *would*, just pretend for the moment that you wouldn't), and you will teach yourself to not go to bed without learning something new.

Third, impress your colleagues. This isn't about competitiveness. It's about competency. It's a lot more fun and gratifying to go to work knowing that you are doing a good job and on top of your game, rather than just "getting by" or "surviving." Learning a little every day, slowly but steadily, will give you a large advantage over your colleagues who are not doing the same. Soon, you'll realize, "Hey, I really get this." And, that's fun—or at least more fun than perpetually asking, "Will I ever get this?"

A last thought on reading: I want to emphasize that I wouldn't advise trying to read too much every night. Having said that, if you want to read a lot in one night, of course do that. But don't use the excuse of reading a lot on one night to mean you don't have to read the next night. Learning a little every day will soon add up to a lot. Make it a daily habit to read at least a little. Habits are hard to break.

👍 DON'T WRITE PRESCRIPTIONS FOR NURSES, FRIENDS, OR ANYONE ELSE WHO ISN'T YOUR PATIENT

When you get your medical license in the state of New Jersey, as I did, you have to attend a series of lectures on your responsibilities as a physician in the state. One of the lectures I attended was particularly sobering. The speaker was an attorney for the state whose job it was to prosecute doctors. She related the following incident:.

A nurse working in a hospital was asking residents for a prescription for Oxycontin. She would tell the resident that she had knee pain or some other ailment and she couldn't get a doctor's appointment for another two weeks. She just wanted a prescription to hold her over until she could see her doctor. The residents, each one apparently hearing what sounded like a very reasonable story, would write her the desired prescription. Because this nurse was only getting one, or at most two, prescriptions from any one resident, no resident got suspicious.

But someone did. Somehow, the pharmacist, the insurance company, or the police (I forget how exactly she was found out) made a phone call. She was investigated, and her whole scheme came tumbling down. It turned out that she had been selling the drugs on the street for a sizeable profit. The residents were hauled before the state medical disciplinary board.

 LESSON LEARNED

Imagine that—having just received your license and having to go before the disciplinary board to face possibly *losing* your license because you tried to help out a coworker who seemed to be in pain. All of this before even graduating residency. It doesn't seem fair. The disciplinary board took mercy on the young physicians, understanding that they had been duped, and told them to take this as a sobering learning experience and to be much more careful in the future.

Another story from a community hospital told by a different source with a more devastating ending follows.

A resident wrote a prescription for Ambien for a unit clerk who said she had been having trouble sleeping. A few weeks later, the unit clerk didn't come to work. When she did reappear at work, she was in a leg immobilizer. She said she had taken the Ambien one night and gotten up, felt dizzy, and fallen in her bathroom. She had dislocated her hip. The unit clerk held the resident who had prescribed her the Ambien responsible. She sued. When the lawyers asked to see the resident's medical records on the unit clerk, the resident had to explain that the clerk was not really his patient.

"Of course she is," the plaintiff attorney insisted. "Doctor, you wrote a prescription for her. Don't you know that once you write a prescription for someone, that person is automatically your patient? She is just as much your patient as if you had been treating her in your own practice. Now, I'll ask you again, doctor, where are your records?"

The resident lost his medical license and was suspended for a year from his residency. I don't know what ultimately happened with the lawsuit. I was told it dragged on for a while and that the resident who was in the hospital at the time moved on. In any case, the result could not have been a good one. I also don't know whether the hospital's insurance would have covered the resident for writing the prescription, because that wasn't part of his hospital duties.

Here's another story, in case the point has not been driven home yet. This one isn't about an intern or even a resident. It is about a family practice doctor in an affluent suburb in Florida.

A family practice doctor was making rounds in the hospital. A nurse he had known for more than 10 years approached him complaining of a sore throat. Strep throat had been going around, and a few of the other nurses were already out sick with it. The doctor looked in her throat and diagnosed her with strep. He told her that he could get a swab and culture her, but really she should just take some amoxicillin. The doctor wrote the prescription, and the nurse was very grateful. The nurse turned out to be allergic to the antibiotic.

She had a reaction and ended up in the hospital for a couple of days. She sued.

Here is one final story on the subject. This one was also told by the attorney at the lecture to the young New Jersey doctors.

The attorney was talking about the dangers of writing prescriptions for family members. She said that it was not uncommon at all for husbands and wives to write each other prescriptions once in a while. But, she strongly cautioned against this. For one, she argued, it was probably not good medical care. For another, she said, on multiple occasions, during or after a divorce, as a form of revenge, the person who had been treated as a patient had filed a complaint with the state medical board about inadequate medical care from his or her spouse. When the board went to investigate, as they are required to do following such a complaint, they inquired about the doctor's medical records.

The husband or wife would say, "What medical records? She was my wife!" Or, vice versa— "He was my husband! I didn't keep any medical records." This is unacceptable, the attorney explained at the lecture. If you write a prescription, that person—wife, husband, grandparent, or child—becomes your patient. And, any patient must have a medical file to document your diagnosis and treatment plan. No exceptions. To not have documentation on your patient is malpractice and can lead to suspension or termination of your license. Moreover, it is certainly an excellent platform from which a lawyer can build a juicy malpractice suit if so inclined.

LESSON LEARNED

Before I had my license, I remember calling a friend who was an attending physician. I asked him for a simple prescription for an antiinflammatory drug for a friend. The physician said he would be happy to write it, my friend just had to come in for a visit. "It doesn't even have to be a formal visit," he told me. "I can see him after hours, whenever is convenient. And I won't charge him. I just have to be able to lay eyes on him and create a file on him before I can prescribe any medication."

At the time, I was put off by my attending physician friend. It wasn't that he was disagreeing with my diagnosis or that he thought it was the wrong drug to give. He just wanted to cover himself medicolegally. Today, having gone through the process of getting my license myself, I completely understand where my physician friend was coming from.

Once you have your medical license, it's *yours*. It is your responsibility to safeguard it. Once you get your license and can write prescriptions, people will ask you for things. "Doc, can you just write me a small script for Ambien?" "Hey, doc, remember me? I've got a sore throat. Can I have an antibiotic or something?" Et cetera.

I strongly advise you to set your limits early. Make clear rules for yourself and then do the hard part—follow them. Remind anyone who says that you're not being "flexible" that it's *your* license. Even a close, old friend can have a bad reaction to a medication. And, that friend can have second thoughts about how close the two of you are. Incidentally, your friend would be right to be angry with you if you prescribed a medication without really doing a full exam and work up and a bad reaction occurred. That is, after all, shoddy medical care, and you'd be doing your friend or relative a disservice to "treat" him or her. Friends, family members, and associates who aren't doctors don't realize that it's not appropriate for you to write a prescription if they aren't your patient. They don't realize that it is suboptimal care. They think that you can diagnose them over the phone or at a dinner party just as you could in the office, and they don't realize that you could lose your license for doing so. Will they feed you and your family if you lose your job and license? If there is an adverse event, the patient doesn't even have to sue for you to get in trouble. One of the ER doctors might ask who made the diagnosis and who prescribed the medication. The charges can start that way.

Each of you is naturally going to decide for yourself how you want to handle the new responsibility of being able to hand out prescriptions. If you do treat family members or friends (and I'm not recommending that you do), I implore you to at least treat them as you would any other patient. Take a history, do a physical exam, and be sure to create a medical record. The medical record is there in case something happens and also for future reference and management decisions just as you would have for any other patient.

KNOW THAT AT TIMES, YOU'LL HAVE TO FORCE YOURSELF TO STEP IT UP A NOTCH

All through life, as you know, you come to moments when you have to manage your fears and self-doubts, maintain your composure, and do something that you are afraid to do or don't think you are able to. These moments might include when you had your first success with toilet training . . . were dropped off at school to face the world without your parents for a day . . . first told a bully that he couldn't have your lunch money . . . first asked a girl for a date . . . learned calculus . . . first moved away from home . . . cut into your first cadaver . . . and so forth. These are all crossroads, of course, which everyone deals with differently. As an intern, you will come to many such crossroads: telling someone his or her loved one has died, running a code, or answering your page when you're bone tired in the middle of the night, and going to see the patient even though you just want to give an order over the phone.

I am reminded of a pep talk that one of my soccer coaches gave before a big game. The big game, for us, at the time, was a crossroad. Would we step up and bring our game to the next level? Would we choke under pressure? Our coach looked at, and into, each one of us and said, "These guys are bigger than you. They're stronger and faster than you, and they've played together longer. No one thinks you have much of a chance. But they don't have something you do. Something they can't touch, and they can never take away. They don't have your heart. Go out there and show them what that means."

During my third-year medical school medicine rotation, I gained the trust of my resident. He and I felt confident that I understood the basic management of most of the pathologies we were treating. I learned to write comprehensive notes. One day, the intern on my team was off at a meeting. My resident said to me, "I'm going to do something for you. It'll be a good lesson." He picked up the phone and signed my intern's pager into my own. Then, he gave me his password for the computer. (A disclaimer: Remember that one of my previous pieces of advice was to never give your computer password to anyone. This rule still applies, and this story in no way mitigates that.) and told me to take care of any issues that came up on the floor. "It's pretty quiet today. You'll be fine." He would be in the library if I needed him, he told me.

I was sure he was joking until he got up and left. Then I felt numb. What if someone called? What if someone needed something? Medical students at that hospital didn't put in orders (especially since it was a computer order system), and I had never written an order of my own command. Occasionally, on other rotations, I may have written the occasional order when directly told what to write by a resident or attending. This was different.

For a while, I felt nervous carrying the pager around. I kept looking at it. Finally, when an hour had passed and no one had called, I began to like it. I felt like, well, I felt like a doctor. Besides, I reasoned to myself, I understood what was going on. My rotation was basically done, and I felt that I could manage simple problems. If anything complicated came along, I would call my senior. Easy.

Then, it beeped.

I called the number. "Doctor, are you covering the 4th floor?"

"I am," I told her.

"I have a patient here, Ms. Z. She just came up from endoscopy, and she is complaining of a lot of pain. She doesn't have any pain medications written for her. Her family is at the nurse's station and they're complaining. Can we give her something?"

I was on the 5th floor at the computer station. "Absolutely. I'll be right there," I said. Pain medication. Okay, that shouldn't

189

be too hard. What can I give her? How old did the nurse say she was? I realized I had forgotten to ask. My heart started beating faster as I made my way for the stairs.

I found the patient's chart and scanned through it. A young man, evidently the patient's son, saw me with his mother's chart. "Excuse me, doctor," he said, "that's my mother. She is in a lot of pain. Can we get her something now? She shouldn't have to lie there like this."

I nodded. "We'll get her something right away. Let me just go see her."

I carried the chart as the son led me to his mother's room. There were other family members there. The patient, an elderly woman, was alert but clearly in discomfort. I did a brief exam. "We'll get you something to make you feel better," I told her.

I went back to the nurse's station, still holding the chart. What could I give her, I wondered. At the time, I hadn't done any pain consults, and this was the sort of thing that the intern was called about, not the medical student. No one had ever asked me about pain medications. Still, I thought, Percocet seemed reasonable. Wait! What if she had liver problems? Could I give something with acetaminophen in it? I scanned through the chart again looking for any evidence of liver problems. None were listed, but it didn't look like anyone had checked her liver function tests. Could I give her acetaminophen without knowing if she had liver problems? Why not just give Advil? No, of course that wasn't strong enough and, anyway, what if she had stomach or kidney problems? Why not give her some oxycodone? But how much? She was a little old lady. What if I gave her too much and she stopped breathing? What was a small dose for someone of her size and age?

I had always written medications on my notes, but I had never concerned myself too much with actual dosages. I looked it up and 5 mg seemed right for her. But how could I be sure? I decided that it wasn't fair for her to wait while a medical student debated this. I called my senior resident, but soon realized that he wasn't calling back. I called again. Still nothing. I was on my own. I saw the son pacing a few feet away. I couldn't blame him. His mother was in pain. All of a sudden, a small panic set in. I knew I should have been able to give something easily. I felt that I could offer three or four very reasonable alternatives, but which was the right one and at what dosage? What if I were wrong and something bad happened? Should I have this much responsibility as a 3rd year medical student? Was that fair to her?

Finally, I saw an attending I knew. I told him the story of the patient and asked whether 5 mg of oxycodone sounded right. He agreed and so that's what I gave.

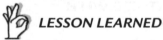

LESSON LEARNED

In the years to come, the feelings I experienced and the thoughts I had in those 15 to 20 minutes are almost comical to me. But they served an important lesson. In those 20 minutes, I learned about the pressure that comes when someone else's, a stranger's, well-being depends on *you* and *your* judgment. Giving a small dose of pain medicine during internship quickly became an easy task. But, during internship, life and death decisions are frequently made. Sometimes, you are the most senior person there, and you have to make the call. Starting internship is like starting anything else in many respects. Your first day of internship, you don't know that much more than you did on your last day of medical school. Of course, in internship, the learning curve is steep and unforgiving. Hence the crossroads.

The world is stronger, less forgiving, and a lot older than any of us. It has chewed up and spit out people far smarter and more studious than you and me, and it hasn't experienced any remorse about it. As you step into your role as a doctor—a role coveted by many and granted to few—I remind you that there will be doubts. Always act in the best interest of your patients, and always get help or ask advice when you are unsure. But I beseech you, when the time comes for you to step up, always remember to stick out your chest, show what you're made of, and bring your game to a higher level.

REFLECT UPON HOW YOU FEEL DURING INTERNSHIP SO THAT WHEN YOU ARE A RESIDENT, YOU CAN EMPATHIZE WITH YOUR INTERNS

For some reason, it seems to me that the residents and attending physicians who have the hardest times during internship seem to be the same ones giving their interns the hardest times later on. I am not sure of the reason for this. It may be that they are angry and frustrated and see this as a form of payback. I don't believe this to be the case, though. I have known several very kind and thoughtful residents who were cold and hard on their interns, and I don't think it was out of spite. It may be that they feel this is somehow a necessary part of internship. Or, perhaps they are having a harder time as residents and attendings and thus feel the need—conscious or subconscious—to vent some of their fears and frustrations on their most vulnerable underlings. Whatever the reason, I think this kind of passed-down abuse wouldn't happen nearly as much if people would just pause during internship, and again during residency, and remember how it feels to be an intern. Remember how overwhelming it can be and how many indignities are suffered.

A more benign example of the above is the following:

A friend of mine had a very difficult internship. His wife told me on more than one occasion that he was considering quitting his program. Fortunately, he stuck it out and went on to enjoy his residency and currently is thriving in private practice. When we sit and talk about the past, he tells me that actually his internship really "wasn't that bad."

Wasn't that bad? *I am always amazed when I hear him say that. When I remind him how bitterly he complained, how he considered quitting on multiple occasions, he shrugs it off as if it never happened. In his case, as a resident, he was not cruel to his interns.*

LESSON LEARNED

I know several instances similar to that offered above. Probably, not remembering how bad an experience was once we have finished it is a healthy human survival technique. Perhaps, this helps women have second, third, and more children after a difficult labor. Whatever the reason, it's a natural and very prevalent phenomenon. You probably have done it at some point in your own life. My first day of going to high school? It wasn't that bad. I was a little nervous, but not much. Preseason training? It was fun. I mean, yes, it was tough and Coach could be a pain, but overall, it wasn't all *that* hard and we had a good time. Medical school? Not bad. There was a lot of studying and it was stressful at times, but we still had fun.

Very few of us have the ability to remember our past events and our emotional reactions to those events with detachment and accuracy. It is far easier to sugar coat the past. Again, this is probably a healthy thing to do. Who wants to think that life has been tough? Who wants to remember and relive pain? Especially if everyone else is saying that something wasn't so bad, then it probably wasn't so bad for you, either. So the process feeds itself.

I would urge you to do the same for internship, except that this has the potential to make you cold and indifferent to the suffering of future interns when it is their turn. Instead, yes, remember the positive moments, but also remember the sleepless nights, the fear, the anxiety, and the abuse. No, internship isn't *all* bad, but don't forget that it isn't all good, either. Hold on to how you feel going through the process, so that you will have the appropriate empathy when it's your younger colleagues' turn.

REMEMBER HOW LUCKY YOU ARE TO BE WHERE YOU ARE

When I started medical school, our dean told us a story during our white coat ceremony. He told us about how talented our class was and how *lucky* we were. For every one of us, there were equally or more talented candidates who had applied but weren't accepted into medical school. Aside from a few geniuses scattered here and there, there are more talented people than there are positions in medical schools. And, for internship and residency, there are again more talented people than there are spots. Most of us are lucky to be where we are. Of course we worked hard, of course we think we "deserve" it, but our colleagues who weren't as fortunate also worked hard and also deserved it. We don't need to feel guilty about that. We should just recognize our luck and let it help keep us humble.

👍 REMEMBER THAT IT'S ONLY ONE YEAR!

At times, internship can seem endless. Long hours, more stress than you have ever had to deal with, life-and-death decisions, sleepless nights—it is a difficult year by all accounts. But, when it's all said and done, you do learn a lot. And, despite how it may feel at times, it is just one year. I hope this book helps, and I wish you all the best in your present and future endeavors.

Index